S0-APN-029

Caring Comes First

Caring Comes First

The Story of
The Leprosy Mission

Cyril Davey

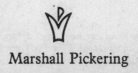

Marshall Pickering

Marshall Morgan and Scott
Marshall Pickering
3 Beggarwood Lane, Basingstoke, Hants RG23 7LP, UK

Copyright © 1987 Cyril Davey
Front cover photography by Ursula Sadie,
courtesy of The Leprosy Mission
First published in 1987 by
Marshall Morgan and Scott Publications Ltd
Part of the Marshall Pickering Holdings Group
A subsidiary of the Zondervan Corporation

All rights reserved. No part of this publication may be reproduced,
stored in a retrieval system, or transmitted, in any form or by any
means, electronic, mechanical, photocopying, recording or otherwise,
without the prior permission in writing, of the publisher

British Library CIP Data

Davey, Cyril
   Caring comes first
   1. Leprosy Mission
   I. Title
   362.1'96998   BV2637

   ISBN 0-551-01434-2

Text set in Plantin by Brian Robinson, Buckingham
Printed in Great Britain by Hazell Watson & Viney Ltd,
Member of the BPCC Group, Aylesbury, Bucks

For
LUCY and PHOEBE

Contents

Foreword

There was one firm instruction from the International Director – and it was the only one he gave me.

'Always avoid the word "leper"!'

Except where it could *not* be avoided, in quotations for instance, in the early sections, the instruction has been followed. It is not a touchy or pernickety 'mission attitude'. 'Leper' is universally recognised as an offensive term, banned by governments and the World Health Organization for some forty years. It degrades people who have a disease that does not kill, is not infectious in the same way as flu or a common cold, and cannot be caught by touching someone who has it. But, because for centuries it has caused terror and revulsion, those who suffer from leprosy have been rejected by society. Even to use the word 'leper', however ignorantly or innocently, is to make a man or woman feel less than human.

A century ago, when The Mission to Lepers in India was slowly emerging as a caring Christian society, no one thought of the word as being hurtful. But in that century everything has changed out of recognition. The pivotal point of transformation was only forty years ago when four words flashed round the world that were to bring new hope and life to leprosy patients and workers alike. *Leprosy can be cured!*

This book, which it has been a privilege to write, tells the story that led up to that point of change, and what has happened afterwards. It is, in fact, *two* stories. One is the story of what is now The Leprosy Mission International. I have been captivated and humbled as I have exposed the drama, the dedication and the faith that lights up the whole of that story. It cared when almost nobody else cared for leprosy sufferers. The first part of its 'objects' was 'to minister in the name of Jesus Christ to the physical, mental and spiritual needs of leprosy sufferers' – and for more than a century it has never failed to put caring first. But that work of compassion can only be fully understood against the background of the struggle with leprosy, and so the two stories have been told in tandem, as it were, though coming ever closer together as the years pass. As it unfolded I began to realise that there is no other drama – and in particular no Christian story – quite like that of The Leprosy Mission. But someone else will have to write the final chapters, for the struggle and the mission still continue unended.

From the beginning I have had the fullest possible help from The Leprosy Mission and I must record my gratitude to two of its senior officers, Eddie Askew and Bill Edgar, and my indebtedness to Elizabeth Harland for constant practical help. The list of materials used and consulted, mostly from the Mission's own shelves, is much too long to quote but quite invaluable.

I hope the conviction will grow in you, as it has done in me, that the Mission's founder spoke the simple truth when he said, 'This is a work of God!'

Prologue in Berlin (1904)

The Fifth International Dermatological Congress, meeting in Berlin, was thronged with medical and scientific personalities from all over the western world, enthusing and arguing in a dozen languages. Professional expertise was everywhere. 'Herr Doktors' and 'Herr Professors' jostled at every corner, and there certainly seemed no place for non-scientific amateurs.

Yet the quiet Irishman who stood up to face the distinguished gathering had no qualifications whatever, and he was announced by the President merely as 'Mr Wellesley Cosby Bailey from Scotland; the Secretary of The Mission to Lepers in India'. He at once made it plain that he had no competence in medical matters – though he did express his pleasure that the First International Leprosy Congress meeting here in Berlin seven years earlier had insisted that leprosy was a contagious, not an inherited, disease. This statement was in line with his own conviction which had deepened with the years and had shaped his own Mission's long standing policy of segregating healthy children from infected parents with notably good results. For the rest, his address was a factual account of the rise of the Mission and its work, colourful with stories of the rejected sufferers to whom the Mission had brought hope, comfort and faith.

At the end of his talk doctors, scientists, research workers and university professors rose to give him a prolonged ovation, clapping until the President turned to the surprised Irishman.

'You have done more for the lepers in India, Mr Bailey, than all the doctors and scientists together,' he said. The applause was renewed until the speaker had left the platform.

It was an extraordinary moment.

What had this one-time missionary done to deserve such a tribute from such a gathering? Certainly nothing to advance scientific knowledge about leprosy. But in the thirty years since he first saw leprosy sufferers huddled outside their huts at Ambala he had – without deliberate planning, though he believed with the help of God – created and maintained a Mission which, by 1904, had an annual income of some £50,000, all of it given away in small sums to assist churches and missions in their own compassionate work for people with leprosy. He had seen that work extend throughout India and to Burma and China.

What Wellesley Bailey and his Mission offered to people with leprosy was no more than compassionate care – food to eat, medication to alleviate ulcers and burns, acceptance instead of rejection, hospitals or leprosy homes overflowing with love. Or so it must have seemed to those who came to them. However, the workers themselves knew there was more than this. There was the compulsion that drew them into the work – the gospel of Jesus Christ who loved the sick and the whole, the seeker and the sinner, and who seemed to have a special concern for those whom other people despised.

What he had done gave grounds enough for men of science to write an accolade to Wellesley Bailey in the Proceedings of their Congress. In Asia disabled people would have expressed their response in a different way. They would have bent to touch his feet with their clawed hands.

Wellesley Bailey had, in fact, done considerably more than was apparent in thirty years. He had begun to accumulate a fund of compassion. He had made an increasing number of people in Europe and America aware that leprosy was not a half-forgotten phenomenon of Bible days but a devastating disease of our own times. He had preached everywhere that Christians had an obligation to succour those who suffered from it now, in their own time. With a growing if still small band of like-minded, concerned men and women, most of them declared Christians, he had begun to change the emotional climate. If leprosy sufferers were to be helped it would not be because people's minds were alerted to new facts but because their hearts were touched.

1: The Fight Against Leprosy: The Living Dead

When and where did leprosy begin?

Nobody really knows. Archaeology has not produced evidence of its existence in primitive times and the first clear and accurate description of the disease is found in India about 600 BC. It may well have been carried from the east by international travellers. It was noted in Greece in 300 BC where it was called both *leontiasis* because of the lion-like appearance it gave to the face, and *elephantiasis* because it caused grossly swollen legs. The armies of Alexander the Great returning from Asia may have brought it to the eastern Mediterranean, while the Roman legions may have been carriers to Rome and Gaul, spreading it through northern Europe. To the Iberian peninsula and Britain the carriers may well have been Phoenician tin-traders. By whatever means, leprosy had spread across Europe by the time Christianity was established there.

The Bible, in its English translation, refers to 'leprosy' in Old Testament times – far earlier than that first Indian description. Authoritative writers on leprosy, however, supported by most biblical scholars, believe that the word which sixteenth-century bible-translators rendered as 'leprosy' really meant something completely different, both in the Old and New Testaments. Depending on circumstances it could well have been any of several unpleasant and contagious diseases, and this equally applies to the leprosy-sufferers in the miracles of Jesus. Certainly the 'white-all-over' patches drawn by biblical illustrators do not represent leprosy! The confusions were accentuated because in the sixteenth and seventeenth centuries the English word 'leprosy' was used to describe a wide variety of diseases such as scabies, tuberculosis and syphilis which could easily be caught by close contact.

It is historical fact that by Wycliffe's time, and certainly when Coverdale and the King James translators were at work, true leprosy had almost entirely disappeared from Britain and most of western Europe. It is also true that for a thousand years or more leprosy had been a prevalent scourge in Britain and Europe. Those who suffered from it had been condemned to a living death. They were isolated but even then, all too frequently they were attacked and murdered.

This episode from the Middle Ages may seem barbaric to twentieth-century Christians but evidence for it is built into the lovely gothic parish churches all over Britain – the so-called 'leprosy squint-holes' through which the leprosy-sufferer outside the church could stand and watch the priest at the altar as he celebrated the mass. This must have been a painful reminder of the last time he or she had been inside a church themselves. On that occasion he – or she – had been hustled into the parish church for a dreadful service of expulsion. Sex and age, like the deformities the disease had produced, were hidden under a black cloth. Sometimes the leper would stand, shrouded under the cloth, in front of the altar. At other times he would crouch under two trestles with a cloth flung over them – the trestles on which a corpse was normally laid for a burial service. He would then hear the priest say 'the mass of death' – that is, read the burial service over him and scatter earth on him as he would over a corpse in an open grave. For all real purposes the person with leprosy was now dead to society. Led to the church door he must stand and listen to the list of prohibitions. He may never again enter a church, a house, a tavern or a market-place. He may not walk through narrow lanes or speak 'down wind' to anyone he passed. He may never speak to children and must always wear a 'leper's uniform', though its colour and design would vary from place to place, with gauntlet gloves. He must always give warning of his approach either with a bell or more frequently with a rattle.

This indeed was 'a living death' for thousands of people in mediaeval Europe.

At times, too, the death might not be symbolic but real for, when society became particularly frightened that leprosy was spreading, sufferers might be attacked and cudgelled to death. Even worse, as too many records show, the sufferer might be buried alive.

However, the Church was also known to show mercy. All over Europe 'leper hospitals' and 'lazar houses' were opened by monks and nuns to care for those whom church and society had rejected. The 'lazar houses' derived their name from St Lazarus – though no one could ever be certain whether he was the man with leprosy who sat at the rich man's gate in Jesus's parable, or Jesus's own friend Lazarus who was raised from the dead.

Both religious and civil attitudes to leprosy shifted unpredictably. When Crusaders who had fought to regain Christ's tomb from the Saracens ended up bringing back leprosy from the Holy Land the Church proclaimed that they should be honoured because they were sharing the sufferings of Christ himself. Yet, in 1340, Edward III ordered all persons suffering from leprosy to be clear of London in fifteen days; after that, if they were found in the city, they would be killed.

Then, for no obvious reasons, leprosy in England halted its advance and began to recede, and after the fourteenth century 'true' leprosy almost completely disappeared.

Folklore, on the other hand, maintained the popular superstitious dread of a disease few people had ever encountered. So, in the last century, did Sunday school teaching and Bible picture books. Even today, for people ignorant of the true facts, leprosy remains mysterious and terrifying. At the same time, the terror that had prowled through mediaeval Europe was no mere nightmare story in Asia and Africa. It was *real*, the appalling daily condition of millions of people.

In the last century no one had any idea how many in India or China had leprosy – but everyone thought they knew where it came from. The answers varied from religion to religion. It was a curse from the gods; a man's *karma*; the result of sin in some past incarnation; the inscrutable will of Allah or the sign that the spirits of the ancestors were angry. Many believed it was passed on from one generation to another.

The signs of leprosy could be hidden for months or even years under a dhoti or a sari but they would eventually give place to more visible manifestations – fingers and toes would begin to curl up; hands would lose their sensation, and so would other parts of the body; faces would become disfigured. And because neighbours and even families were terrified that the same thing would happen to themselves if the sufferer remained in close contact with them he, or she, would often be driven out to scratch or beg a meagre living from the hard land or the charitable passer-by.

In Asia, Africa and the rest of the world those who had leprosy often came to feel that they would be better dead. In the 1870s there was no cure for them, no hope, no home, no future.

That was when Wellesley Bailey saw them for the first time.

2: An Irishman in Search of a Future (1846–69)

Gravesend was still shrouded in fog and the young Irishman paced the deck impatiently, listening to the creak of the wooden ship. This was Tuesday, 28th August, 1866 – surely no time of the year to be fog-bound in London when twenty-year-old Wellesley Bailey was on his way to Australia to make his fortune! He had a sudden momentary sense of unease. Australia? Was that where God really wanted him to be? A few days earlier he might not have thought of God at all; now, after the unexpected experience in Gravesend parish church and in his cabin, the question was inescapable. And he could not be certain of the answer.

He wondered what Alice Grahame was doing, back in Ireland.

Wellesley Cosby Bailey grew up at Abbeyleix, Queens County, in southern Ireland, in a spacious Queen Anne mansion. His father, hard-riding and, on market days, hard-drinking, was agent for the Cosby family estate and the Baileys were sufficiently well-off to send their four sons to a boarding-school in Kilkenny. Wellesley was a careless scholar, more interested in horses than books, and in later life he insisted that his own children's considerable abilities came from their mother and not himself. Though living in deeply Roman Catholic country the family worshipped at the Church of Ireland but in church, as at school, the boys' thoughts always wandered to far-off lands. When they left school Wellesley's brother Christopher went into the

Indian army and Alfred joined the Carbiniers. This urge to travel was hardly surprising. Ireland, in the 1840s, had been plunged into the dreadful potato famine and, with North America and the colonies seeming to offer the only hope, over a million people emigrated from Ireland in the late 1840s. Twenty years later Wellesley Bailey followed the same pattern, setting out to find his fortune in the newly-developed goldfields of Australia. Only saying goodbye to his boyhood girlfriend Alice Grahame made him hesitate – and that not for long. He was too young to be tied down to a woman, and he sometimes wondered whether, in any case, Alice was not a bit too religious for someone as volatile and adventurous as himself.

At last, with the sails hoisted and the ship slipping down the Thames, he said farewell to England and saw Gravesend slipping into the distance, the parish church still rising above the roofs of the quayside buildings.

Because the ship had been delayed by fog, and because he had promised Alice Grahame that, though he did not share her Christian faith, he would go to church when he could – and perhaps most of all because he had only just left behind Ireland and all he knew – he had gone to Gravesend parish church the previous Sunday. In the service he had felt a sense of Christ's presence such as he had never known before and, in his own cabin, on his knees, he had committed himself to God for the rest of his life. For ever afterwards he would be Christ's man. Now, setting sail down the sluggish Thames, his future was in Christ's hands.

Three years later, docking in Dublin, he felt he had wasted three years of his life. He had failed to find gold in Australia. He had been disappointed when he tried stock-riding in the farmlands of New Zealand. New Caledonia, in the Pacific Islands, proved even more disappointing. Disillusioned, he had set sail for Ireland, asking God what he should do next.

God's answer seemed to be provided almost as soon as he reached home, for his brother Christopher wrote from his

Indian army station suggesting that he come out and join the Indian police. Wellesley took to the possibility at once. He was always eager, ready to respond to a new challenge – and perhaps India was where God wanted him to spend the rest of his life. In 1869, aged twenty-three, he sailed away once more, to make a future in the Indian police service at Faizabad where his brother Chris was stationed.

By the time Wellesley reached India, however, Christopher had been moved to another station on the North-West Frontier and Wellesley found himself in totally strange surroundings, overwhelmed by the noise, the heat, the flies and the vividness of the bazaars, his ears battered by unfamiliar languages – and he was gripped by the country and the people from the moment he arrived. Faizabad, in what is now Uttar Pradesh, was a busy administrative centre as well as a holy city and a place of pilgrimage. Not far away was Ajhodia, one of Hinduism's most sacred shrines where the great god Rama had been born.

A future in the police seemed to slip out of his mind. Surely there were more constructive things he could do – beginning by studying Hindi. In order to do so he lodged with Mr Reuther, an old German Lutheran missionary working with the Church Missionary Society, in a mission-house made out of a deserted Muslim memorial tomb. He also met regularly with a group of Christian soldiers from his brother's regiment, and began to learn the craft of public speaking in their meetings and Bible classes. More important, from 'dear old Mr Reuther', as he described him, he 'received his first drawings towards missionary work'. Now, at last, the path ahead seemed clear. He had worked – briefly! – in the Pacific; he had had good schooling in Ireland; most important he had a firm faith. Very little more was needed for a missionary teacher and the American Presbyterian Mission accepted him for one of their schools in Ambala.

There, in the Punjab, he settled for the first time in his

life to steady, disciplined work in congenial surroundings with people who were totally committed Christians. The leader of the mission in Ambala was a very able and distinguished American minister, Dr J H Morrison, who soon came to like the enthusiastic young Irishman, and Wellesley, busy teaching 400 children during the day, was quickly immersed in other areas of Christian witness and service in the evenings and on Sundays. From conversation in the mission he heard, in the phraseology of the time, that 'Dr Morrison looked after some beggars who were lepers' but even after a few months he had no idea what this really meant. Conditioned by Bible stories like Naaman the Syrian commander-in-chief, he had a mental picture of men whose skins were covered with scaly white areas. Then one day Dr Morrison suggested he should visit the beggars' huts with him.

'I have been caring for forty beggars with leprosy. Nobody else wants to do anything for them but I've built them some huts where they can have shelter. There's no hope for them, of course!'

It was a cool December day in 1869, with bright sun and clear skies, when Wellesley set off with Dr Morrison – and found himself crossing the road, only a little way from their own compound, to three rows of small, rough huts under some trees. Outside were gathered a group of people, waiting for worship to begin. Staring at them Wellesley realised he had seen people exactly like them without realising what or who they were, thrusting begging-bowls at him in the bazaars with mis-shapen hands. These, then, were sufferers from leprosy – quite unlike his Sunday school picture of them! Some had hands with the fingers permanently clawed inwards; some seemed half blind; others had disfigured faces. The children, on the other hand, seemed perfectly normal. Dr Morrison watched him, wondering how he would react to his first sight of this rudimentary leprosy asylum.

'I almost shuddered,' Bailey wrote afterwards, 'yet I was

at the same time fascinated, and I felt if there was ever a Christlike work in the world it was to go amongst these poor sufferers and bring them the consolation of the gospel.'

There had been a number of false starts but at last Wellesley Bailey, the young Irishman, had found his future.

3: Unexpectedly, in Dublin (1869–75)

When Dr Morrison, who was unwell, had to take local leave in the hills he had no hesitation in handing over the leprosy work to the young newcomer who was showing such unexpected interest in it. What revolted most westerners – and that included many missionaries – Bailey found a compulsive challenge, though he saw his mission at first as being specifically evangelistic. His Hindi was becoming rapidly more fluent and as he talked with them he discovered the outcasts' reason for the despair which showed so often in their faces. They believed their leprosy was a curse from the gods, and this became the springboard for his talks with them as he squatted outside their huts. If their own religion rejected them because of the gods' displeasure, Wellesley Bailey welcomed them into the Christian family because Jesus loved them. It was a very simple gospel, proclaimed in hesitant words, but to Bailey's joy some of the hopelessness was dispelled as a few of the beggars were baptised into the Christian community.

Then, like the gentle St Francis many centuries earlier, Bailey realised that preaching was not enough and when he discovered that other missionaries were involved with leprosy work he began writing to them to find out what they were doing.

At the same time Wellesley Bailey had another correspondent, and a very different reason for writing. In 1870, by sea-mails that took months to travel to and from Ireland, he became engaged to his childhood girlfriend Alice Grahame, and his letters were no doubt properly romantic. But they were also filled with stories about his leprosy work and those parts of them, at least, Alice shared with her friend the Pim sisters in Dublin. They overflowed with questions and problems, too. He was already asking where leprosy really came from, whether it was contagious or hereditary, whether little children might be exempt from it if they were kept away from their parents. Why did some sufferers lose all sensation in fingers or feet, others produce dreadful ulcers, and yet others have no more than pale insensitive patches for years? More urgently, what could be done to ameliorate their sufferings?

Some of the answers to his own questions began to appear in his letters. He was finding that other people besides Dr Morrison had shown practical concern. As long ago as 1812 William Carey, the pioneer Baptist missionary, had seen a man with leprosy buried alive and had been stirred into opening 'asylums' in Calcutta and Allahabad which were still there. A young army officer, Ensign Sir Henry Ramsay, had set up an asylum of his own at Almora, and that too still existed. Nearer at hand, at Subathu in the Simla hills, an American Presbyterian missionary, Dr John Newton, had built huts, as Morrison had done at Ambala, for leprosy sufferers – though his main problem was finding money to support the work.

Describing it all to Alice, Wellesley said leprosy sufferers' 'first and greatest need is the gospel, but in taking them the gospel it soon became evident that a good deal more was needed; eg good living rooms, good food, clothing, medical attention, sanitary regulations, etc, and that much more could be done for them along these lines.'

All this concern and compassion Alice shared with her Dublin friends the Pim sisters, Isabella, Charlotte and Jane, before she said goodbye to Ireland and sailed for India. Met in Bombay by Wellesley, still as exuberant as she remembered him, they were married in Bombay cathedral, travelled north by slow trains over the flat brown landscape until they reached Ambala and were shortly afterwards transferred to another Punjab garrison town, Ludhiana. Alice brought to this new partnership many of the qualities her husband lacked. Like him her speech was unmistakably Irish and they both radiated charm, conviction and compassion but Alice was restrained where Wellesley's enthusiasm ran away with him, and persuasive where he was sometimes vociferous. She was an excellent musician, playing the piano and violin, and a notable linguist, adding Punjabi to her fluent French, German and Italian. Many of her academic and artistic gifts she passed on to their four children, one of whom was to become a teacher in India and then a professor at the School of Oriental Studies in London. Yet Alice always regarded her truest task as supporting her husband and, in time, providing a full and family life for their children.

Sadly, two years after her arrival in India it was clear that Alice's health was not standing up to the excessive dry heat of the Punjab and it was agreed that the Baileys should resign from the American mission. They were then sent back to Ireland. This was a deep disappointment, though it meant that Alice did recover her full health. Then, in September 1874, came a decisive happening. Their friends the Pim sisters invited Wellesley and Alice to stay with them in Dublin and then asked Wellesley to talk to a few friends in their drawing-room in Alma Place about his work with the leprosy sufferers in India. He proved so enthusiastic and interesting, and the whole subject was so new, that a more public gathering was arranged in the Friends Meeting House. At this meeting Wellesley again described leprosy to people who hardly knew that it still existed; spoke of the sufferers in Ambala whom he had helped and talked of Dr Newton's work in Subathu limited only by lack of funds. He stated, 'For as little as £5 an adult leper can be cared for in an asylum, and a child for much less than that.'

The same challenge was issued more widely in print

when Wellesley's afternoon talk was produced in booklet form, a minuscule tract, only a couple of inches square, containing sixteen pages. Entitled *Lepers in India* it quickly sold out and was to be reprinted again and again. It was to be the essential tool in a campaign launched as the Pims and the Baileys walked home from the Meeting House that afternoon.

Charlotte Pim spoke hesitantly. 'I think we could perhaps raise £30 a year for these poor people. It is not much but . . .' She saw the look on Wellesley's face. 'If you are now going back to India you would be able to put some of it to use yourself!'

With Alice now fully recovered Wellesely had managed to obtain an appointment with the Church of Scotland Mission which sent them back to India. They sailed in December and were posted to a missionary station in a small hill state, Chamba, lying on the borders of northern India and Kashmir. And, by the time they sailed, some three months after Wellesley's talk in Dublin, it was clear that his words and the Pim sisters' enthusiasm had started a fire that would not be put out.

Charlotte's promise of 'perhaps £30 a year' had been startlingly transformed into an actual cash sum of over £600 by the end of the year. With extracts from his booklet and from his letters reprinted in the mission's magazine Bailey's work became more widely known and contributions came in ever more quickly and generously to Charlotte Pim who had readily agreed that she would handle the money and send it on to India.

There was no society, no organisation, no committee. But, quietly and unexpectedly that Sunday afternoon in the Dublin Meeting House, something had begun which would not be destroyed by disappointments, false starts, even two world wars . . . something which would help to bring new hope and new life to millions.

4: The Fight Against Leprosy: The Great Discovery (1873)

In September 1874 Wellesley Bailey had been assailed with questions in the drawing-room at Dublin when he had talked about leprosy. 'What *is* leprosy? How is it passed on? What causes it?' He replied quite simply: '*I* don't know. And *nobody* knows!'

But Bailey was wrong. In the previous year, 1873, a Norwegian, Armauer Hansen had discovered the cause of leprosy. Leprosy had much the same history in Norway as it had in the rest of Europe. Viking marauders, bringing back Irish girls from their raids, apparently brought back leprosy with them, too. As it had done in Britain the disease spread, was treated in the same desperate way and, by the fourteenth century, had begun to die out – except in one place. Even in the nineteenth century the countryside surrounding Bergen had an appallingly high level of leprosy but in Bergen itself, where probably three people out of every hundred suffered from it, the authorities, instead of driving them out, built rough-and-ready hospitals in which they were isolated from the rest of the community. In 1839 Daniel Cornelius Danielssen, one of the earliest leprosy experts, was put in charge of Bergen's Lungegarden hospital.

He began working in the white-washed, timber-framed hospital with a colleague, Carl Wilhelm Boeck, and together they started to try and define the disease which had baffled people for centuries. In 1847 the two doctors produced an epochal book titled *Om Spedalskhed*, or *On Leprosy*, which for the first time provided a clear, scientific presentation of the disease in its two main forms. The book was based on detailed research carried out on the corpses of patients who had died of leprosy. This research always had to be undertaken in shrouded rooms at night, by the light of lamps and candles, to avoid the anger of fellow townsmen who believed the trolls would take vengeance on anyone who tampered with the dead. Danielssen's investigations showed that seventy per cent of his patients came from families with a history of leprosy and he drew the not surprising conclusion that leprosy was an inherited disease. It was the outstanding error in his immensely distinguished career.

Gerhard Henrik Armauer Hansen was born in Bergen in 1841, when Danielssen had been at work in the leprosy hospitals for a decade, and choosing medicine as a career he went to work with the great leprologist. He never forgot his first leprosy contacts in the hospitals, or his sense of outrage at the deformities leprosy caused and the resulting sense of exclusion from society. Leaving Norway to pursue his studies he went first to Germany and then to Vienna but, back at last in Norway with fresh enthusiasm and knowledge, he plunged once more into research work under Danielssen. He was then just over thirty, some five years older than Wellesley Bailey.

With Danielssen he concentrated attention on one particular phenomenon the older man had originally noted under the microscope – the yellowish-brown, frogspawn-like masses in the biopsies taken from leprosy patients. There was never anything different in the thousands of specimens they examined, yet Hansen had an intuition that, though their research remained stagnant, the secret must eventually be discovered under the microscope.

On 28th February, 1873, Hansen brought into the laboratory two biopsies which he had obtained from the nose of one of his patients. For the first time he noted, within the granular spawn-like mass, a host of tiny rod-shaped bodies like tiny sticks. There were hundreds of these microbes to be seen.

Armauer Hansen had discovered the bacillus which was soon to be accepted as the cause of leprosy – the *mycobacterium leprae*. This discovery was the first time a bacillus and a disease were clearly linked with each other, and represented a leap forward, not only in the fight against leprosy but in medical science and the treatment of disease.

Scientific research, of course, seldom runs smoothly and Hansen faced all sorts of problems and criticisms. Danielssen refused to back down from his own position that leprosy was hereditary. Hansen in turn, was involved in court cases because of his experimental work with patients in the hospitals. A German who had come to study under him returned home to claim that *he*, not Hansen, had discovered the bacillus. In time, however, as tensions eased Hansen's reputation mounted steadily and he was to be acclaimed throughout the world as the greatest of all leprologists.

In 1909 the Second International Leprosy Congress was held in his own home city of Bergen and Hansen himself was appointed to preside over it. He was fêted, acclaimed and applauded. But this Congress, like the one in Berlin a few years earlier, had one remarkable feature. Hansen himself had invited Wellesley Bailey, the sixty-year-old non-professional ex-missionary to share fully in its work – a tribute not merely to a great man but to the compassionate work of The Mission to Lepers in India and the East.

In 1909, thirty years after Hansen's discovery of the leprosy bacillus, loving care and a tender welcome were the only things that could be offered to the millions of people who suffered from leprosy throughout the world.

5: The Making of the Mission (1875–86)

Wellesley and Alice went back to India in 1875, knowing nothing of Hansen's important discovery of the leprosy bacillus but well aware that the support in prayer and money of friends in Dublin would enable them to do *something* for the leprosy sufferers they met. Problems arose out of the fact that by now Wellesley was a lay-missionary of the Church of Scotland whose task was evangelism, not dealing with leprosy and he was finding it difficult to know what practical action he could take under this new brief.

The difficulty the Mission had with Wellesley Bailey was his enthusiasm! He toured the Himalayan foothill state of Chamba, sharing his own love of Jesus with ebullient fervour. He planned to open a boys' school in the city and wrote to Edinburgh about establishing a chain of schools in hill-villages, but he had a chilly reply. 'One *good* school is more use than a dozen poor ones!' Leprosy remained on his mind everywhere he went. Only a few months after he arrived in Chamba he wrote to Charlotte Pim. 'I have been on tour and find that leprosy exists to an almost appalling extent!' Later, he wrote again to acknowledge the gifts she had sent from Dublin. 'I have built eight huts for the lepers in Chamba.' The first entry in his cash-book was: '5 annas to coolies for marking the site' of the 'leprosy asylum' which friends in Ireland had made possible. The second entry was, in a sense, more significant. '1876: 1st June. Sent to Subathu – 400 rupees.' That first gift from Ireland he used for work other than his own. Wellesley's Subathu

31

association had begun some years earlier on his first trip to India when he had come to know Dr John Newton, minister and doctor of the American Presbyterian Mission. Newton had established a 'poor house' at his station in the Simla hills. Now, knowing the Baileys were back in India – but ignorant of what had happened in Dublin – he wrote to share his frustrations. A woman who had tramped and begged her way through the Himalayas for ninety miles, disabled with leprosy, had been the first occupant of his new poor house; now there were more and more clamouring for help, many of them with leprosy and he could neither take them in nor, in conscience, drive them away. Bailey's response of sending 400 rupees from Ireland was an astonishing answer to prayer that would be repeated hundreds of times in the years ahead all over India and beyond.

Two events in Chamba substantiated Bailey's conviction that God had called him to demonstrate Christ's compassion to those who had leprosy. One was the arrival of the first gift from any overseas church, a small amount given by Bailey's own congregation, themselves desperately poor. The other happening was in the leprosy huts he had built. One of the earliest sufferers to be accepted was a Muslim, Rasullah. When the disabled man was told that he was going to die the news gave him only joy. Rasullah was one of the first converts of Bailey's compassionate leprosy work and his words were memorable. 'I am ready. Whether I live or die my trust is in Jesus the Lord'.

Unaware of the research in Norway, which for many years would have no practical effect in the leprosy hospitals, the workers in India and elsewhere kept on asking the same question. 'Is there *no* way the disease can be halted?' And, from Subathu, came what seemed like a message of hope.

When Dr Newton went on leave his place was filled by Bailey's old chief from Ambala, Dr Morrison, and Morrison wrote to Bailey saying he had heard from an old friend, Dr Doughall. Doughall was the medical officer in the penal settlement in the Andaman Islands and he had found, by accident or experiment, that gurjan oil, extracted from trees native to the Islands, had an ameliorative effect on convicts suffering from leprosy. Bailey, in response, ordered a fifty-gallon cask of gurjan oil to be sent to Morrison at Subathu. Full of hope, it was applied to residents in the poor house – but whatever the result in the Indian ocean it did no good in the Simla hills. It would be only one of a continuing number of false hopes.

The Dublin cash-book had another entry, in the long run far more important than the abortive expenditure on gurjan oil. It was a gift of £240, a very large sum in the 1870s, to the Rev J. H. Budden of Almora specifically for work amongst children.

Bailey was already strongly convinced that leprosy was infectious, not hereditary, and that intuition was shared by the Budden sisters and their brother, the Rev J. H. Budden of the London Missionary Society working at another asylum. Their special contribution to leprosy policy was to separate children from infected parents before they themselves contracted the disease. The results were encouraging. Healthy children brought up in a separate home on the same compound as their parents did not as a rule develop leprosy and the policy of separation was later to become basic to The Mission to Lepers in India.

At this stage, however, there were only the Pim sisters and their helpers, receiving and responding to enquiries, letters, promises and gifts. And though Wellesley Bailey was half a world away he remained a very effective advocate of the leprosy cause in Ireland and Scotland. Soon after he and Alice returned to India there was issued the first of a long series of half-yearly *Occasional Papers*, quoting from his letters and descriptions, and including lists of donors. His minuscule book, containing Wellesley's address at the Dublin Meeting House, went through reprint after reprint and was quickly known, from its price, as *The Penny Beggar*. The Church of Scotland in its mission magazine reprinted stories from all these sources so that more and more gifts reached Dublin.

There still existed the problem of how Wellesley could reconcile his ministry to lepers with his original brief given by the Scottish Mission, which was to evangelise, rather than to heal.

The Mission headquarters in Scotland had agreed that Bailey might 'work with the lepers if his proper work does not suffer', but in reality matters were not as straightforward as that sounded. What *was* his 'proper' work? Untrained, except by experience, he went on teaching, preaching and evangelising – but he could not shut his eyes or his heart when he saw someone suffering from leprosy. At the same time, some of his colleagues on the field, like members of the board in Scotland, were clear about one thing: 'The Irishman isn't paid to work with people with leprosy.'

The truth, of course, was that no one anywhere was 'paid to work with people who have leprosy'. Everything that Morrison, the Buddens, Newton and the rest did was *extra* to their 'proper' work, a voluntary service in love for the rejected. If Christian missionaries did not care for them it seemed no one else would do so. Not only were missionaries not paid to do this work; no missionary society or board carried any responsibilities in their budgets for it. Leprosy sufferers were at the very bottom of the heap when people in need were discussed. Apart from a few caring individuals and those whom they had set on fire with their own passion it had not yet occurred to any Protestant church or charitable group that somebody should do something about leprosy.

Even in Dublin, where Charlotte Pim spent much of her time dealing with correspondence and money, the situation was formless and haphazard. Could Wellesley Bailey, she wrote, come home, just for a month, to get things on a proper footing? Reluctantly his Mission board gave permission after three years' service for a month's leave, though they made it plain that these divided loyalties could not be tolerated much longer.

It was only on Wellesley's return to Ireland in 1878 that The Mission to Lepers became properly formalised. The Committee of The Mission to Lepers in India was appointed and officers elected, with Charlotte Pim as Secretary. She informed the new committee that they were raising about £900 a year and Bailey reported that they were assisting and caring for about a hundred leprosy sufferers, mostly in North India. Wellesley Bailey was appointed the first Secretary and Treasurer, to work from India. A new Mission had now officially been born and was ready to step out in effective action.

The next period began, and continued, uneasily. In 1879 the Baileys with their children were back in India. As unpaid Secretary for India Wellesley was caught up in increasing correspondence. Requests for help had all to be investigated and reports sent back to Dublin, and this took time. Tensions increased with some of his colleagues. The Mission board was uncertain where to station him and then, once more, Alice's health broke down. In 1882 the Mission Board ordered them home and took them off their missionary lists. Wellesley was once more without any paid employment.

It seemed as if he was still in search of a future as he approached his forties, a married man with three children and with eleven years of missionary service to his credit. It would, in fact, be yet another four years before the pattern finally took shape and he moved fully into the place for which God had so evidently been preparing him. For the moment he became Secretary of a Scottish mission working among women in India. In 1882 the family moved to Edinburgh which was to remain their home through the long years ahead.

In his new appointment he was permitted to spend time on the affairs of his own Mission as one of its two

Secretaries, the other being Charlotte Pim. Indeed, he spent so much time and money on the work that he was three years later granted £30 a year for expenses! The income increased, but so did the requests for help. In India his old friend J H Budden had taken his place as the Mission's Secretary for India and, forwarding the policy of creating compassionate homes and refuges, he sent an increasing number of requests for finance. A year or so later Mr Budden attended the Dublin Committee and reported on all that was happening.

'So many things have changed, in so many places the work has grown, in so many other places things are happening that even we in India do not know about them . . .' He urged that Mr Bailey should tour the whole of India and see for himself what needed to be done. 'The headquarters of a Mission should be in touch with what is happening on the field . . . and this *is* the Mission to Lepers in *India*!'

In 1886 Wellesley Bailey at last moved into his proper place. Giving up his post in the Scottish Zenana Mission he was appointed the full-time Secretary of The Mission to Lepers in India, although the Committee was based in Dublin – it was very much an *Irish* society for the time being – and the Baileys continued to live in Edinburgh. For the moment that hardly mattered. Early in that same year, 1886, Wellesley and Alice Bailey set off to visit India. They did not return to Scotland until the spring of 1887.

6: The Fight Against Leprosy: The Hero of Molokai (1889)

A Norwegian, an Irishman and a Belgian were the key-figures in the struggle against leprosy which began in the latter part of the last century.

And, for each of them, 1873 was a crucial year. In the over-all purposes of God these three great men, unknown to each other and unsuspected by the rest of the world, were used to focus knowledge, concern and emotion on those who suffered from a disease which more than any other isolated them from family, local community and society as a whole.

It was the year Hansen discovered the leprosy bacillus.

It was the year Wellesley Bailey first visited the leprosy huts in Ambala.

And it was the year the Belgian priest, Joseph de Veuster, sailed from Honolulu to Molokai, the island of death. Sixteen years later he himself died there.

When he died only a small number of medical pro-fessionals understood the work Hansen was doing on the leprosy germ, and there were still comparatively few supporters for The Mission to Lepers in India. In contrast, the death of Father Damien – the name by which he became known – amongst men and women living in a tainted island gave rise to a surge of worldwide interest, compassion and activity. Not only did it stimulate Christians to new endeavours but it stirred those with influence and authority into action. The 'leper' – and no one had yet used a less-loaded word to describe the sufferer – was until then a 'creature' who was less than human. The influence of Father

Damien was to begin to transform such sufferers into real men, women and children. It would be a long road before the very word 'leper' was recognised as derogatory and would be outlawed – but the journey had begun.

Joseph de Veuster was a Belgian peasant with all a countryman's characteristics. He was vigorous, tough, practical and obstinate – all qualities he would need in full measure. He entered the priesthood in 1860 and when his brother, designated for the Pacific, developed typhus he wrote and offered to go in his place. He never saw his parents again and served as a parish priest in Honolulu for eight years ... until the day the bishop, Monseigneur Maigret, dedicating a new church, spoke about Molokai, an island to which anyone with leprosy was exiled for life. No visitors were permitted – and now the government had even forbidden the priest to visit it and offer the consolations of religion.

Impulsive and easily moved Father Damien stood up after the sermon and offered to go to Molokai, to live and die there. He had little opportunity to change his mind. There was a boat due to sail from Kohala to Molokai, with leprosy patients aboard, in a few hours time. On that May day, 1873, Father Damien sailed with them.

The situation on Molokai was appalling. Drink and sexual licence were the only release for people who were there until they died. There was no fresh water, no sanitation, no decent housing, no self-respect. Decomposing corpses lay here and there, unburied. Slowly, Father Damien began to change things – until, in time, he changed everything. He started burying the corpses with his own hands. He walked the hills until he found a fresh-water spring, and piped it down to the plains. He imported wood for proper housing; began schools; built a church; and then more churches throughout the island, filling them with men and women who had come to love him, and to love God through him.

At last, after more than ten years, came the terrible and

dramatic day. Damien had always begun his homilies at Mass with the words 'My beloved brethren . . .' Now, on this morning, the words were changed. He looked at the congregation bearing so many signs of leprosy and began to speak. 'We lepers . . .'

After fifteen years visitors were allowed on the island to see and write about the transformation. A few others came to stay, and serve. Damien's story began to circulate the world and when, on 15th April, 1889, Father Damien de Veuster died, the conscience of the world began to stir. It was moved even more by an open letter from Robert Louis Stevenson who had been to Molokai. Here and there groups and individuals offered money and service.

In Britain there was a royal response for at a great meeting in the Royal Albert Hall the Prince of Wales himself was the main speaker. A campaign to 'eliminate the foul disease from the world' was set up – the National Leprosy Fund – and in the following year a Commission (the fourth since 1850) was sent out to make a survey of leprosy in India.

By the time the Commission returned Wellesley Bailey had himself toured India with his wife, surveying what the Mission was doing and what more needed to be done.

7: '. . . and the East'
(1886–93)

The cost of a passage to India in 1886 and a 9000-mile tour within the country was by our current standards a very meagre sum – very fortunately since the annual income of The Mission to Lepers in India was about £1000. It is notable that no record exists of anyone questioning the necessity of such visits; the work of the Mission depended for many years on Bailey's own knowledge, gained at first-hand, and passed on in his own talks and writings.

This first tour took the Baileys from Bombay to Bengal, from South India to the North-west Frontier. Wherever he went Bailey made careful notes on institutions run by missions, private charity or local government. He knew precisely what he was looking for. 'In my experience, now extending over a considerable number of years,' he wrote 'I have found the inmates require good food and clothing, kind medical care, plenty of fresh air, room to move about, good bathing accommodation and something to occupy their minds – light gardening, or learning to read, or something of that sort.' It was all a long leap from his own first experiments. His criteria were far ahead of his time and were by no means generally met. At Pallypuram hospital, with a foundation stone dated 1728, there was no one in charge at all. At Alleppey the sufferers 'lay uncared for on a sandy floor, their untreated ulcers a horrible sight'.

There were, of course, more encouraging visits to Christian missions which would in time become splendid institutions linked to Bailey's own Mission. One of these was Purulia. At this town on the Bengal border a charitably-minded District Officer had once built a few rough thatched huts for the leprosy-beggars who ranged the bazaars. His successor, seeing them as a public nuisance, had burned the huts and driven their inmates out of town – but not for long. They drifted back, went on begging, and lay out in the open ground where their huts had once been. A German missionary, Heinrich Uffmann, had written to Bailey asking for support if he began an asylum and now Bailey, leaving his wife in better comfort, set out for Purulia – a train from Allahabad; a midnight wait for a *palki*, a manhandled litter sent by Uffmann; a bumpy ride in it until the following midnight and then, at last, Purulia. Over the following days he and Uffmann sought a possible site and discussed the future. At that stage Bailey imagined that £100 a year should be sufficient for its maintenance, but could have no idea how absurdly inadequate his own estimate would be!

Wherever they went on this and following tours Bailey was treated as the expert. Because leprosy work was always an unsupported extra to a mission board's programme he was not only the adviser, but the only source of financial aid if his ideas were to be followed up. Though the money he could provide was usually small such assistance could mean the difference between continuance and closure of work begun, and was frequently the first step to long co-operation. Alleppey in the south, which Bailey had found so depressing, and Purulia and Naini Tal in the north, all visited on this first tour, were to become important homes and hospitals linked with the Mission.

This first tour included one other significant visit – to Government House in Calcutta to meet the wife of the Viceroy of India, Lady Dufferin. It proved no mere viceregal gesture. 'Her Excellency was most kind; much interested in hearing of our efforts and had visited the Leper Hospital in Madras' he later wrote.

Returning to Scotland by mid-April 1887, Bailey

reported to his Dublin Committee that he had visited over twenty institutions aided by the Mission as well as many that were not. But if their Committee were to carry the weight needed for its future work and influence it must be considerably strengthened – and he had some daring suggestions. They must have sounded grandiose to the little group in Dublin – but the Anglican Archbishop of Dublin agreed to become President and the Marchioness of Dufferin and Ava, the Lady Vicereine, the Patron of the Mission. That, however, was not enough to guarantee the support the Mission needed, in spite of a number of new ventures. Three widely-scattered 'auxiliaries' had been formed in England (though most of the support still came from Ireland and Scotland) at Brighton, Cheltenham and Bolton and Altrincham. Bailey's new book, *A Glimpse at the Indian Mission Field and Leper Asylums*, was unlikely to reach people unaware of the Mission. What was needed was something that would call the world's attention to leprosy and the plight of those who suffered from it.

When Father Damien died on Molokai in 1889 the world was, indeed, shocked into awareness of the needs of lepers and The Mission to Lepers in India shared in the response. Amidst all the emotion other stories reached Britain, and America, notably the account of a woman – hero of the leprosy world. Her name was Mary Reed. She had contracted leprosy and had chosen to bury herself in the high Himalayas to serve men, women and children in the hills who also suffered from leprosy. Concern began to show itself in pounds, shillings and pence.

In 1889, the year of Father Damien's death, the Mission's income was £1,628. However, Bailey calculated that if they were to do all they wanted their income must rise to £5,000 per year. Bailey's seemingly impossible target was reached three years later and a considerable thrust toward it came in May 1890 when the Mission's first public meeting in London was held in Exeter Hall, the rallying-place of English evangelicals. The small audience was enthusiastic and there were two statements from the platform which were widely reported.

The first was from Wellesley Bailey himself. 'I have had letters in the last few months asking us to commence work at nine new centres.' One of these was at Neyyoor in Travancore, South India. There, a London Missionary Society doctor wrote that he had been followed for six miles along a country road by a man with leprosy asking for relief and could do nothing to help. Later, another eight men had come with the same plea, and he could only make the same answer. A grant had been made, reported the Secretary, but much more needed to be done.

The second challenge came from the chairman of the meeting. 'Mr Bailey says we need £1000 at once. I will gladly give £100 if nine other gentlemen will do the same!' It was a speech that guaranteed headlines and as a result a Leprosy Home and a Healthy Children's Home were built and opened at Neyyoor, and one of the Indian medical evangelists being trained at the hospital put in charge. Neyyoor was, in time, to become one of the Mission's most significant centres.

The same meeting heard of another surprising development – not only a new place but a new country. 'We have had an appeal, amongst those nine I have mentioned, for help to begin a new leprosy centre at Mandalay – in *Burma*!'

Burma had recently been added to the British Empire, and British soldiers were quartered in Mandalay. Seeing a new opening for the gospel in this Buddhist country the Methodist Missionary Society sent W R Winston from India as their first missionary – and one of Winston's first activities was to drive round the city in a cart drawn by a distinctive white bullock, looking for leprosy sufferers whom he could care for. Mandalay Buddhists were astounded. Why should a foreigner want to care for people who were painfully working out their *karma*, their deserved fate, from previous incarnations? The house was built with money from the Mission, and the number of occupants quickly grew from fifteen to fifty.

The Baileys were soon to see the Mandalay home for themselves on their next tour and on the same visit helped an American missionary to find a site for a home in Moulmein. At the Committee which followed the tour Bailey's report was even more expansive. 'Now, in 1891, we are responsible for maintaining seven centres; we give two-thirds of their support to three more; eight others are helped to a considerable extent ... altogether we are assisting thirty institutions. .... The Mission to Lepers in India has moved forward very quickly indeed.'

It had moved so quickly, in fact, that it had outgrown its name. Not only was it giving help to Burma. China was asking for assistance too.

It became The Mission to Lepers in India *and the East*.

8: Man on the Move (1893–1906)

There is, of course, no doubt that today's great Leprosy Mission owes its existence to one man, even though he was always eager to give much of the credit, very rightly, to Charlotte Pim who from the beginning maintained the Dublin headquarters and continued this side of the work until her death in 1913. Wellesley Bailey was physically sturdy, with immense reserves of energy. He loved travel, and crammed into his journeys intensive investigation and memorable personal contacts. He was easily liked because he genuinely cared about the people he met and worked with. He never lost the sense that God's hand was on his shoulder, that God directed what he did or planned. The whole range of leprosy care, for him, was sustained because it was God's work.

His tours were not only, therefore, opportunities to see what was being achieved or needed to be done; they were filled with occasions of witness. Travelling widely in India, speaking in Hindi or Punjabi, or waiting while his soft Irish speech was translated by a local missionary, he talked always about Jesus and his love. These were not words that died in the summer heat; they were substantiated by the work of Christian men and women, missionaries and nationals, who welcomed leprosy victims without condescension and with love. Adventurous, highly individualistic and irrepressible, still only fifty, Wellesley Bailey not only felt that God had placed him where he was; he had no intention of delegating his responsibilities to anyone else.

The Commission to India, set up after the Albert Hall meeting, had encouraged him by visiting all the Mission's institutions and had reported in high praise of their work. Meanwhile, his new book was selling well.

To both Bailey and his supporters one proof of the Mission's significance was that it was extending not only in China but into Japan.

A Scotsman, Dr Duncan Main of the Church Missionary Society, on furlough from Hangchow in China, heard of the Mission for the first time and visited Bailey in Edinburgh. 'I've no room in the hospital for these people with leprosy who come to me for help, but I'd like to help them.

'I need £200 to put up a building for the men, and another £50 a year to keep it going. If I'd known about you earlier I would have written to you!' Dr Main got what he asked for, and back in Hangchow wrote a letter of thanks – and rather more. 'By and by you must build me a small place for women ... but of course you would have to increase your annual grant too'.

By the end of the century grants were being made to Swatow, Pakhoi and other China stations.

Then, from Japan, Miss Riddell of the Church Missionary Society wrote to Dublin. Based at Kumamoto, on the island of Kiushiu, she found leprosy sufferers visiting the Buddhist temple, a couple of miles away, praying and hoping for miraculous cures which could not happen. The Christians could not offer a cure, either, but they could provide compassionate care if they had the money for buildings and maintenance. The Mission's response was almost immediate: 'Kiushiu, Japan: for buildings: £200'. Less than a year later, in November 1895, the Leprosy Hosptial at Kiushiu was opened on four acres of ground. 'It includes a house for men,' wrote Miss Riddell, 'a home for women and children, a larger building containing the consulting room, dispensary and waiting rooms, kitchen and offices; then there is a house for the superintending doctor, a bath-house and a *godown* (storeroom). The first patient is a Christian official, the second a Christian school-teacher, the third a carpenter who is not a Christian.' It was a remarkable beginning to notable work in many places in Japan.

The last decade of the century saw the Baileys travelling constantly both east and west. In 1892 Wellesley toured the United States and Canada for the first time. The next year he was invited to Chicago to speak at the World Congress of Missions, for The Mission to Lepers had become an acknowledged component of the Protestant missionary scene. And not only of the missionary scene, for 1897 was the year Wellesley was invited to deliver a paper at the prestigious First International Leprosy Congress in Berlin.

Between Chicago and Berlin there was for Bailey yet another tour of Asia, covering 23,000 miles in six months.

It was the 1892 North American tour, however, which was to have a result at that time quite unimagined. In Canada, at Guelph, Ontario, Wellesley was asked to come back and tell them more before he returned to Britain, and so he did. Mrs James Watt and her daughter Lila organised a drawing-room meeting in their home which led to the foundation of the Canadian Auxiliary of the Mission, and brought a young man of great potential ability face to face with Bailey. The young man, William Henry Penny Anderson, plied the speaker with questions – but neither of them could possibly have looked into the future and realised that Anderson would, in some twenty years time, be Bailey's successor as Secretary of the Mission!

The man who would be used to bring Anderson into the Mission's service, John Jackson, only joined the Mission himself some eighteen months after Bailey's visit to Guelph. He organised a monthly prayer meeting in the YMCA in London for the work of the Mission, which was, however, poorly attended, and a keen disappointment to Jackson even when Wellesley Bailey himself came from Scotland to speak at it. It had remarkable results, nonetheless, for Bailey invited him to work for the Mission, at first alongside his normal business commitments and, later, full-time.

'John Jackson,' said Bailey, 'was one of the greatest gifts God ever gave to the Mission.' He worked for it and in it for twenty-three years; visited Asia, America, Canada and the Pacific; spoke widely and well; wrote articles and books with considerable effect; and organised, quite separately from the Mission, a Missionary Pence Association which eventually became the All Nations Christian College. Before his death in 1917 he saw the Mission's annual income rise from £5000 when he entered its service to £40,000, and its work extend to eighty-seven centres in twelve countries.

However, all these remarkable advances were far in the future when Wellesley Bailey came to the Mission's Committee in 1898. He had a clutch of letters in his hand. 'All these are requests for help. All of them *deserve* help. But we've not only used up our current funds, we've used our reserves, too. We can't do anything new until we've got more resources for the things we're already committed to.'

'Not even for Miss Harvey?'

'No! Not even for Miss Harvey!'

Rosalie Harvey's story was well-known to the Committee. Working in Nasik, in the Bombay Presidency, she was a Zenana Bible and Medical missionary who cared for unwanted children and ill-treated animals, and now wished to do something for the leprosy beggars sleeping on the verandahs of a riverside temple. Miss Harvey's letter was colourful and deeply moving – but nothing could be done.

Or was that really so? Might not an answer lie in using the new magazine, *Without the Camp*, which had begun publication two years earlier? An appeal, specifically for Miss Harvey's projected leprosy work, was included in the magazine and the result was immediate. Miss Harvey had the money she needed. The Mission was on the move again with a new and powerful medium for its appeals.

By 1906 when Wellesley Bailey set off with his wife for

another essential tour of the east he was celebrating sixty years of adventurous life and the Mission was just over thirty years old. But despite all its growing resources it could only offer loving care. Not healing, or even the hope of healing.

9: The Fight Against Leprosy: Segregate! (1889–1914)

How many people suffered from leprosy? Wellesley Bailey's estimate of 250,000 in India at the time of the Commission's visit was grossly inadequate. Thirty years later the 'guesstimate' for India was 'over a million', and that, too, was far below the real figure. However many there were, the urgent problem – if there were no possibility of a cure – was: how can it be prevented from spreading? Since it was increasingly accepted that leprosy was a contagious disease the answer seemed clear: to put those people who have leprosy where they wouldn't infect others. *Segregate them!*

The government of India's 1898 Leper Act decreed that beggars with leprosy should be treated as if they were criminals requiring compulsory segregation from society, and district magistrates were given powers to commit them to authorised establishments. After considerable discussion it was agreed that Purulia, the institution founded by Heinrich Uffmann, would accept sufferers, acting as an institution under the act, though its management firmly refused to accept them if there were any suggestion that they had come under government compulsion. Decisions and control were left to the hospital's own Christian leaders.

What was life like there? Though Purulia was much bigger than most asylums its lifestyle and daily discipline and routine was much the same as in many of the Christian hospitals and refuges maintained or assisted by the Mission.

Purulia began when Heinrich Uffmann, of the Gossner Lutheran Evangelical Mission, returned from his first leave in Germany in the 1880s. His daughter Maria, like her six brothers and sisters, had been born in India but, unlike any of the rest of the family, she had contracted leprosy. Left behind in a Berlin hospital, she died when she was thirteen. Back in India, Uffmann wrote: 'I shall never turn away a leper who comes to me for help.' Nor did he. He gave space to sufferers from leprosy, accepted those whose huts had been burned down by the authorities, took yet more of them into his improvised housing, sought and gained help from Wellesley Bailey on his first tour and, in 1888, opened the Purulia Leprosy Hospital. It was to remain one of the great establishments of the Mission, which supported it through the years, though Uffmann was always needing more and more money to meet his ever-growing number of patients.

The first patient accepted was a fifty-year-old burnt-out leprosy 'case'; a Hindu named Sidham Hinduar. Fifteen months later he was baptised Christaram, won to Christ by the love of solemn, square-bearded Uffmann who, in German-accented Bengali, told him the story of Jesus. When Christaram died they found a surprising poem which he had written. Its last three lines, in translation read:

. . . he is near, with mighty power to save.
His endless grace to sinners has brought life;
Victory is his; he's triumphed o'er the grave.

Uffmann's motive in serving leprosy sufferers was the compassion derived from Jesus Christ himself – and it was Christ whom he wanted, more than anything else, to share with these poor people. If no one could give them healing, Jesus could certainly give them eternal life, as Christaram came so quickly to believe.

When Christaram died there were ninety-nine patients. By 1896 there were 366 – and no room to expand because the municipal authorities of Purulia were increasingly uneasy about the growing mass of 'segregated beggars' on the township's doorstep. Not all, of course, came because they were ill; there was a tendency for the number of patients to show an increase whenever famine left the people on the edge of starvation, and Uffmann's charity was very large. Uffmann, searching for expansion, took over an unclaimed area of jungle a few miles outside the town and with the help of his patients, began to clear away the scrub, dig clay, burn bricks, erect cottages, lay out gardens, build a dispensary, and then, naturally, a chapel. In 1897, when they moved into the new asylum there were 440 patients; by the next year, 527; and in 1900, just over 600.

The Victorian word 'asylum' was inadequate, just as the word 'patient' was misleading. The place was really a new village, with forty three-roomed cottages. Each cottage appointed an elder and the elders controlled the life of community as they met in the *panchayat*, the counterpart of the old five-elder village-council. In the dispensary nurses dressed the patients' ulcers and wounds but, for the rest, dealt with the typical sicknesses of an Indian village. At the single village shop a ration of rice was distributed at the beginning of the week as well as an allowance of sixpence per man and rather less to each woman, and there was new clothing twice a year.

The days were regulated by the chapel bell, summoning those who wished to worship at 7.00 in the morning and again in the evening. There were two periods of preparation for Christian baptism and an hour or so of literacy training. The forty or more children in the Healthy Children's Home had regular schooling and were also taught such trades as carpentry, cookery and housewifery. There was plenty of ordinary manual village labour, too; growing vegetables, cultivating rice, repairing buildings and the rest.

At Purulia, then, as in most of the other hospitals and homes maintained by the Mission, life went on as it did in any other village, and the people who lived there looked like any other Indians – until one saw the clawed hands, the damaged noses and the bandages hiding the rest of their sores.

Outside the leprosy-refuges life went on as usual, too. An unknown number of leprosy sufferers wandered the Indian roads, the forests and the hill-paths and an unknown number of apparently healthy people were in the unseen stages of the disease, unaware that they were passing it on to others.

In the laboratories and research establishments, too, things were normal. Purulia was asked to test an anti-leprosy serum named Leprolin which had been developed by a doctor in the Indian Medical Service but its promising early results proved only false hopes. In the same way there was no future in the Rontgen rays tried out at the Mission's hospital at Dehra Dun or the Nastin injections used briefly at Purulia.

Nothing worked.

The only feasible response to the spread of leprosy over the next twenty years would be segregation.

10: Farewell to the Chief

One March day in 1913 Wellesley Bailey and his wife walked into Waverley station in Edinburgh.

'Yes, sir,' said the booking clerk. 'Where to?'

'Two to Peking. Via Siberia.'

Bailey was now sixty-seven, a little less energetic and tiring more easily, as did his wife Alice. But, as he explained: 'With two weeks on the train across Siberia instead of two months aboard ship, you can get to work more quickly!' He was setting off for the last time to see the work in which he had been engaged for forty years. The Mission was sending him, first, to deal with some difficult situations in China. After that the tour took them on to Australia and New Zealand; through the Philippines, Japan, Korea and back to China; then Malaysia, Singapore and India – sixteen countries; over 150 addresses; constant meetings with officialdom; visits to leprosy homes everywhere; notebooks filled with facts.

Not until April 1914, did they reach London again, but because of fog arrived a day too late to share in the Mission's Annual Meeting. But not even Wellesley Bailey could have dealt with the whole of that tour in one address. It was, in a real sense, the 'Chief's' farewell to the work he had done so much to make possible. That affectionate name by which his colleagues knew him indicated Bailey's position in the Mission and his pre-eminence as a world figure in leprosy work. But it was clear, nevertheless, that he was feeling older – and he already had his eye on his successor.

The first two decades of the twentieth century saw

constant expansion and steadily increased interest and support. Governments had begun to contribute to the costs of the Mission's homes, and were establishing or extending their own leprosy work. A government Commissioner in India reported on a visit to one of the Mission's centres, commenting that it was '. . . essentially Christian but by no means an aggressively proselytising agency . . . moderate in its views . . . liberal in its benefactions' and adding 'I cordially support the recommendation for a grant-in-aid.' In Japan, too, though leprosy work was in the hands of the government and had the personal support of the Empress, the involvement of the Mission was warmly encouraged.

More churches were also offering support. *Without the Camp*, the Mission's magazine, was winning fresh responses to heart-warming, or heart-breaking, stories. The Auxiliaries, or national supporting groups, were growing in effect.

An Irish CMS missionary, on leave in Australia, spoke to a Bible class about leprosy work and so shocked its bank manager leader that he sent an immediate subscription of £100 to London! Eight years later the same man, H J Hannah, was appointed secretary-treasurer of the newly-created Australian Auxiliary. New Zealand, too, formed an Auxiliary. The Canadian Committee continued its task of education and support, and John Jackson – whose business and literary skills had proved invaluable to the Mission – was sent to visit both Canada and the USA, where the first steps had been taken to set up an American Auxiliary. Dr William J Schieffelin, who became its President, was to give such outstanding leadership that the great leprosy research establishment later set up in South India would carry his name.

But John Jackson's visit had a more immediate consequence. In Boston a young chartered accountant, William Anderson, read in the paper that Jackson would speak that night about The Mission to Lepers in India and the East. His mind went back twelve years, to the day he had listened to Wellesley Bailey at Guelph, his home town in Canada. Then, he had been enthralled. That evening in Boston he was moved more deeply and invited Jackson to lunch the next day.

Over lunch he said quite simply that he 'felt a call from God to serve the poor people with leprosy.' Would Jackson accept him for the Mission?

It was not quite so simple, explained Jackson, despite Anderson's evident sense of vocation. The Mission did not send out its *own* workers; it provided support for people in other Missions who were doing leprosy work. He had heard, however, that an American-based German missionary society was having difficulty in finding a superintendent for its home at Chandkhuri in Central India. He suggested that Anderson might perhaps apply to them. For William Anderson that Boston lunch led to the home at Chandkhuri; then to marriage in India; and in 1912 to his appointment by the Mission as its Secretary in India. He served there until 1917 when he was asked to come to Edinburgh.

Amongst those who gave distinguished service to the Mission over this early period was Wellesley Bailey's brother, Thomas, who had often supplied his place in the office when Wellesley was absent on tour. He had worked in homes in India; served as Secretary for the Mission in India; travelled on deputation in Britain and Ireland; visited Canada and the USA; and toured Asia with his wife. The service of such people was greatly important as the calls on the Mission increased.

Many of the new possibilities were in Eastern Asia as well as in India. It is possible to illustrate these growing opportunities only by a few of the calls that reached Edinburgh.

One came, for instance, from Nizamabad in South India. Dr Kerr, the wife of an Irish missionary, was boarding a train when she saw the man who baked their bread – and realised for the first time that he had leprosy. Dr Isobel

Kerr provided him with a segregated hut on their own compound and asked for funds to do the same for other such sufferers. From that act grew the great Leprosy Hospital at Dichpalli which became one of the pioneering institutions in fighting leprosy where it began, in the villages and rural areas.

Another letter was from a woman in Sumatra. This German missionary told a chilling story of a visit to an old woman, condemned to live in a hut away from her village because of her leprosy. 'I got there too late,' said the writer. 'They had burned the hut down that day, and her charred body was still in the ashes.' Four other leprosy sufferers had been killed in that village during the year. With money from the Mission the first leprosy work in Indonesia – then the Dutch East Indies – was begun.

'As far back as 1910 I called attention to the distressed situation of this class of sufferers. As yet not a single effort has been put forth to help them.' So wrote an American missionary, Dr Charles Irwin, from Pusan in Korea. 'I would strongly advise going ahead this autumn with an asylum, and I plan for the support of fifty such sufferers.' Within a year the first Christian leprosy home in Korea was opened – and two more followed in the next seven years.

Another new beginning was in Siam – known now as Thailand – where nothing at all was done throughout the whole Buddhist country for leprosy victims. Then, an American missionary was granted permission to begin work on a conveniently isolated, jungle-covered island in the river near Chiengmai. Again it was the first seed of a remarkable harvest.

The newest ground of all, however, was in Africa. 'Leprosy is a serious factor in some parts of Africa,' wrote a British LMS missionary, 'and I have no doubt you would find a large field waiting for you if you were to begin.' A small grant was made for work at M'berishi, in Central Africa. Africa would never become the major part of the Mission's programme but it would receive considerable help in the years ahead, would provide some of the world's leading leprologists and thirty years later, would be a testing-ground during the greatest single advance towards the cure of leprosy.

Back from their final tour events began to bear heavily on Wellesley and Alice Bailey. Not only did the workload increase every month but some of the Mission's best workers were slipping away. To their distress Charlotte Pim died just before they set off on tour, blind and ill after forty years service in the Mission she had helped to found in Dublin. John Jackson's health broke down and he died in 1917. War had broken out in 1914 and over the following years hundreds of thousands of young men were killed. One of those who died was the Bailey's son Dermot. It was not easy for organisers or supporters to concentrate fully on sufferings far away when those they loved were caught up in the carnage of Europe. For the Baileys the tragedy was still sharper; though they lived in Scotland, Ireland itself was a battleground and their beloved Dublin had fighting in its streets.

In 1917 Wellesley Bailey was seventy-one and in the summer of that year, without private celebration or public fuss, he retired. How did he feel at the end of almost fifty years service in a Mission which still remained the only one of its kind? 'This Mission has been born and cradled in prayer,' he said in almost his last public speech before retirement. 'It has been brought up on prayer; it has been nourished on prayer; and prayer has been at the bottom of its success since the first moments of its life.'

If those were sentiments to be expected of a respected Christian leader were they truly the expression of the man himself? What was he *really* like? Families see people more closely than most observers and a grand-daughter wrote succinctly and objectively about the old man. 'He was not a saint, nor even a clever man. But I do not ever remember hearing from him an ungenerous remark, or seeing him angry apart from minor irritations. His great gift was single-mindedness, and a simplicity that perhaps could not see the difficulties which a more sophisticated mind might see.'

It was a sign of his single-mindedness that he knew just when to retire, and he had no doubt who his successor should be. In 1917 William Anderson, then on holiday in the USA, was recalled to Britain to take his place.

Anderson took over a remarkable inheritance. The Mission that 'was begun, nurtured and continued in prayer' was now helping missionaries belonging to thirty-seven different Protestant societies in twelve countries to care for over 14,000 leprosy sufferers.

It was now a mission with a new name, too. It had become, simply, The Mission to Lepers.

11: The Fight Against Leprosy: The Fruit that Cured the God Rama (1914-39)

The Ramayana is the favourite of all Hindu hero-tales. Played out by puppets, performed by graceful dancers, sung by itinerant minstrels, it is the story of Rama, prince of Ajhodya – near Faizabad, where Wellesley Bailey began his India career – who was banished to the jungles with his wife Sita by the machinations of a jealous step-mother. Sita was kidnapped by Rawan, the demon-king of Lanka, who was only defeated by Rama with the aid of Hanuman, the king of the monkeys, and his monkey army. The little lamps lit all over Ajhodya when they returned home were, in legend, the origin of Divali, the lovely Hindu Festival of Lights, for Rama the prince was to become Rama the god.

Strangely it was this Hindu religious epic that pointed to the first step in the conquest of leprosy.

In 1853 a policeman brought into the Bengal Medical College Hospital a filthy, drunken man who had collapsed in the street. When he was cleaned up it was found he had leprosy. The Indian Medical Service doctor in charge, Professor J F Mouat, was interested in Indian herbal medicine and he remembered an incident in the Rama saga, sung by the street minstrels, which was not often recalled. Rama, then in the jungles, had contracted leprosy but had been cured by eating the fruit of the chaulmoogra tree. There were stories, too, that the fruit had been used for the same purpose in China five hundred years earlier, according to an Indian school-teacher friend of the professor's. He decided to experiment with the remedy himself. He dressed the patient's ulcers with chaulmoogra oil, fed him on pills of the pulped seeds six times a day—and watched the remarkable improvement in his condition until, two months after he had been admitted, the patient absconded, as he said, feeling better than he had felt for years.

All that happened long before the Mission had been established but it seemed that only a small number of interested doctors knew of the incident, though Mouat had sent an account of it to an Indian medical journal and had passed on some chaulmoogra oil to medical friends in Mauritius and China. The articles had not been completely unnoticed, however, for scientists worked on the substance in Paris while in Egypt the Sultan's private physician and a Public Health Officer both proved its efficacy. This last doctor demonstrated it at the Bergen Leprosy Congress which Wellesley Bailey attended, in 1909.

In the Philippines, at Culion, Victor Heiser was creating what was to be the largest leprosarium in the world—made famous by Perry Burgess's notable book *Who Walk Alone*—and there he, too, began to make use of the oil. In every case, however, there was one major disadvantage about chaulmoogra oil. Given by the mouth it produced unpleasant side effects, and by injection it was so painful that many patients insisted they preferred leprosy itself. Nevertheless, it *worked*!

In 1915 Sir Leonard Rogers, one of the medical giants of Asia, was planning to retire after the opening of the Calcutta School of Tropical Medicine which he had spent so long creating. In that year Victor Heiser visited India from Manila specifically to persuade Rogers to delay his return to Britain and introduce the study of leprosy as a special department of tropical medicine. Stirred into immediate enthusiasm Rogers pursued this new work until he retired in 1920 when he handed over the leprosy research department to Dr Ernest Muir, son of a Scottish minister who, since his arrival in India thirteen years earlier, had been concerned with the disease. He was the author of what became for years the standard work in leprosy and was well-known to the workers of The Mission to Lepers. Sharing their compassionate spirit and faith, he was convinced that chaulmoogra oil and its derivatives held the answer to the question they had all been asking. It would arrest leprosy and in many cases would cure it.

After decades of prayer and hard work it seemed that at last asylums and refuges might be transformed into real hospitals offering effective treatment and perhaps sending out people free of the disease that had wrecked their lives.

But if the medical researchers had found a remedy it was not so easy to find the chaulmoogra fruit! True, the trees grew in South-west India, Burma, Siam and Indo-China. But Muir had to find out how and where they could be reached! They ripened in the middle of the monsoon season—and the rains made the forests almost impassable.

One of the most bizarre episodes in the fight against leprosy must surely be the struggle of American botanist, Joseph Bock, and Medical School professor, Ernest Muir, hacking their way through the rain-forests of India and South-east Asia searching for the best chaulmoogra fruit available! That they found it at last, in Kerala, South India, is a tribute to determined courage as well as scientific knowledge.

Sir Leonard Rogers, escaping the heat of India, nevertheless soon tired of England. He returned to India to give his full time and attention to the conquest of leprosy. The Rev Frank Oldrieve was the India Secretary of The Mission to Lepers and a good friend of Rogers' but both of them were aware that much more support could be available for the struggle against leprosy than would be readily given to a western-based Protestant missionary society. With the support of highly-placed government officials in India,

Calcutta businessmen and some of the Indian princes they were able to establish an organisation which is still an influential partner in the work to eradicate leprosy from the world. This was the British Empire Leprosy Relief Association – BELRA for short, and in our own time known as LEPRA – with which Oldrieve and other workers of The Mission to Lepers were at various times very closely associated. Over the next few years other leading figures in the leprosy world moved easily from one organisation to another. Dr R G Cochrane, for instance, joined The Mission to Lepers, transferred to BELRA, went back to Mission and eventually became head of the important Chingleput Leprosy Research Centre, first under The Mission to Lepers and then under Government of India. In all this movement there was no wish to look for greener fields, only the intention to be in the right field of service at the right time.

By the 1930s Rogers' and Muir's work meant that chaulmoogra oil in forms suitable for hospitals and leprosy centres could be marketed at a cost of 2/6d (in present currency, 12½p) for twice-weekly dosage.

The transformation in the leprosy scene between Wellesley Bailey's retirement in 1917 and his death in 1937 was almost unbelievable. Children separated from infected parents could be maintained in health. Leprosy patients could be treated. Most could be helped. Some after a long period, would be discharged 'symptom-free' and – if the community would receive them back – could rejoin their families and villages.

Yet all this was not enough. At the Fourth International Leprosy Congress held in Cairo in 1938 a Christian leprologist whose work in Nigeria was soon to be of great significance made a solemn declaration to which the whole Congress assented.

'It is hopeless to try and control leprosy in a community merely by establishing treatment centres. We are very far from finding a specific cure for the disease.'

The Cairo Leprosy Congress did not know, however, that on the shelves in Germany was a drug which might accomplish much that they hoped for, but which had long been put aside as too toxic and too dangerous for use. Nevertheless, it would still be some years before it appeared on the leprosy scene. For the time being what was still, even in the late 1930s, spoken of as 'the new treatment' – chaulmoogra oil – was offering new hope and new life.

12: Between the Wars

'The new treatment', now available in very inexpensive forms, had undoubtedly brought a transformation to the work of those involved with leprosy, and even more to those who suffered from it. In 1925 the word asylum was outlawed, and replaced by 'hospital' with its promise of treatment and cure – though it still did not occur to anyone that the word 'leper' might itself be an offensive term.

The note of euphoria sounds high in a report by Frank Oldrieve, the Mission's Secretary in India. 'I have visited all the large asylums . . . wherever I have gone there is a different spirit . . . ulcers are being healed . . . faces become normal . . . sensation returning in place of anaesthesia. The hypodermic injection gives no troublesome reaction. Patients are now eager to take the injection and even little children do not dread it.'

Oldrieve was perhaps seeing what he hoped to find – certainly he had not watched the children very closely! – but reports from Japan, Korea, China and South-east Asia as well as India seemed in general to agree with the optimistic tone. As things turned out, the early hopes were not all fulfilled; lepromatous leprosy continued to resist the new treatment. On the other hand, other forms of leprosy *did* respond. Patients *were* discharged symptom-free. The word 'cure' was in wide use, and deservedly so. Though patients did, in fact, hate the injection many of them, after a few years, had no need of it. A story from Dr Isobel Kerr in Dichpalli summed up the changed attitude. 'I noticed a patient was slow in coming forward for his injection, and I asked why. His reply was: "I was saying grace before I received it"!'

The Mission's hospitals existed both to bring healing where

that was possible and always to witness to Christ as the source of health and life. Korea provided one example amongst many of the way the new treatment aided evangelism. Patients were never force-fed with Christianity but a fifteen-year-old boy Oh Sung Soo was happy to attend worship and, in the end, was baptised. This boy had crawled for long days to the hospital after his parents, under threat from their fellow-villagers, had tried to drown him and knife him, and eventually drove him away, daring him ever to return.

After three years he *did* return from the Taegu hospital— *cured*! A few months later a hospital evangelist visiting his village found that Oh Sung Soo had already prepared the way and villagers were eager for the gospel. Within a few months a church was established in the village.

In 1917, when Wellesley Bailey retired, World War I still dragged on in Europe, with appalling casualty lists. In Asia the Mission had to deal with long delays in correspondence, rising costs, shortage of supplies and the internment of German missionaries serving in India – to the distress of the missionaries themselves, the officers of the Mission and the people they had served so lovingly.

William Anderson, who took over from Bailey, was clearly the right man in the right place at the right time. His compassion was matched by administrative ability and financial expertise, and when he moved to the Dublin headquarters he took the first of several dramatic initiatives. They were to include a new address, a new aim and a new policy about missionaries.

The Mission to Lepers was an international organisation and his first reform was to bring the headquarters into an international setting. A delay of eighteen days in a planned trip to America because of misadventure with the England-to-Ireland steamer emphasised what he had long felt – that Dublin was no longer the right place for the Mission Headquarters. The 174th Committee met in Dublin – and the next in London. Though Dublin remained the headquarters of the Irish branch of the Mission, the Mission's address henceforward was in London – first in Henrietta Street and then, for forty years, in Bloomsbury Square.

London was not only the heart of an Empire – the imperial rulers of the 1920s had no idea how soon that Empire would be dismantled – but the headquarters of most of the great British missionary societies with which The Mission to Lepers had such close relationships.

Except for one American woman missionary, Mary Reed, working in the Himalayan foothills The Mission to Lepers had never had a missionary of its own. It had its own institutions but not its own personnel. Instead, it used its steadily increasing income to pay missionaries of other societies who were working in Mission to Lepers institutions, and to support missionaries working amongst leprosy sufferers in homes and hospitals run by other societies. The policy worked well, and Anderson's new initiative was by no means sweeping in its effect. On tour in India the new Superintendent of the Mission heard that the Bengal government planned to collect thousands of beggars suffering from leprosy off the Calcutta streets and put them in institutions. Purulia was one of their chosen centres. If something like this happened new staff would be needed and no other missionary society had anyone to spare. A young man, Donald Miller, who had been discharged from the Royal Army Medical Corps on health grounds, had applied to The Mission to Lepers hoping for an opening with them. After a series of changed plans on the part of the Bengal government, which did not finally initiate its scheme for the beggars of Calcutta, Donald Miller found himself the first missionary actually chosen and appointed by The Mission to Lepers. He was to spend twenty busy years in India being prepared by God for the day when he himself would take on William Anderson's responsibilities and become the third Superintendent of The Mission to Lepers.

Anderson's leadership, meanwhile, between two world wars was a time of change, advance and consolidation. The Mission, which had so far been concerned with amelioration, added a further aim – *to aid in the attempt to rid the world of leprosy*. At the same period the American Auxiliary decided to take on a national identity, and became The American Mission to Lepers, Incorporated.

1924 was Golden Jubilee year and Wellesley Bailey, the Founder, gave thanks as he spoke about years of unimaginable progress under God's guidance and blessing. But there was sadness, too. Alice Bailey, his wife who had shared it all with him, died just before the Jubilee; and so did Jane Pim, who had continued the work in Dublin that her sister Charlotte had begun.

Ten years later, at the Diamond Jubilee, Wellesley Bailey was too frail to leave his Edinburgh home and he died, in 1937, at the age of ninety-one, full of thanksgiving.

During this period new work was begun in the far West in Panama; in Africa; and extended in Asia. Relationships with ruling authorities were generally good, not least in Japan where the work would soon be isolated by war. In Siam (Thailand) the government had once reluctantly found a river island near Chiengmai for leprosy sufferers; now the king and queen of Siam visited the Chiengmai leprosarium to encourage the work. They, of course, were Buddhists but whether it was in Buddhist or Hindu countries the response of visitors was often very much the same, crystallised by a Hindu member of government visiting an Indian hospital: 'This is a wonderful work. Only Christians would show so much love to people such as these!'

There was now much more activity in homes and hospitals than there used to be. Patients were more fully occupied with useful work. Children and young people were busy in their spare time as well as in school. Ten children's homes were founded between the Jubilee and the Golden Jubilee, and Scouting and Guiding were becoming increasingly popular. A report from Cuttack made heart-rending reading. Samviri had had leprosy since she was three and now had no proper feet and no more than stumps for arms. She was bitter, despairing and quite unresponsive. Then one day, she watched a Guide trying to do a knot for her 'tenderfoot' test.

'*That's* not the way to do it!' muttered Samviri.

The girl stared at her. '*You* couldn't do a fisherman's knot, anyway! You've got no hands!'

'Get me a stick and that hook off the well-rope, and I'll show you,' answered Samviri.

Then, with a piece of wood tied to one armstump and a hook strapped to the other she struggled on and on until she had done her fisherman's knot.

It was a new beginning. Samviri joined the Guide company, became one of its outstanding members and was later presented with the Nurse Cavell badge, the Guides' equivalent of the Victoria Cross, for bravery. In time she grew into a splendid Christian woman – the more so, she said, 'because I carry about in my body the marks of the Lord Jesus'.

William Anderson's inter-war years were marked by yet another initiative. New drugs, treatments and hospitals were all signs that the struggle to rid the world of leprosy had entered a new phase. In the past it had usually been adequate for nurses and aides to deal with sores, sicknesses and ulcers; now, *doctors* were needed as they had not been in the past. To meet the new situation a pioneering appointment at headquarters was planned. Dr Thomas Cochrane was a member of the Mission's Council and had conducted a survey in world leprosy. He had also given to the medical world a son more distinguished than himself. Dr Robert G Cochrane had been appointed The Mission to Lepers' Medical Adviser in India in the 1920s and had more lately served with BELRA. Now he was appointed Medical Secretary to The Mission to Lepers in London. It was very much a travelling commission and he immediately set out to grade the Mission's hospitals into A, B or C grades – and went on to work at up-grading those which did not meet his own standards of efficiency and excellence. He proposed scholarships for young Indian doctors who were prepared to specialise in leprosy – and from that scheme came some of the outstanding specialists who served the Mission through the decades ahead.

In 1937, when Wellesley Bailey died, the clouds of war were gathering on the European horizon. Hitler was stridently demanding more 'living-space' for an expanding, Aryan Germany, and proclaiming death to the Jews. But it was in China that the storm broke first and the Mission did not anticipate it any more than most observers in the west. Anderson, not long before, had toured China and visited many of the Mission's notable institutions. In India he planned for the creation of a new home and hospital at Faizabad, which was begun in 1938.

By that year Japan had invaded Manchukuo and begun its ambitious struggle to turn Asia into a Japanese empire. The attempts to keep Chinese leprosy work alive were brave but hopeless for Japanese rule in China was followed by the then equally anti-western communist regime under Chairman Mao. Links between Chinese leprosy work and The Mission to Lepers, severed under Japanese rule and unmended under Chairman Mao are at last being renewed by the much more open current government.

Even in 1939, however, the Sino-Japanese war seemed a far-off localised conflict, unlikely to affect the rest of the Mission's work in Asia. Thailand with its work in Chiengmai, or the hospitals in Burma at Mandalay or Moulmein, seemed safe enough. From Moulmein, for instance, came an encouraging account of a home filled with eager and well-occupied patients. 'Everyone can do something . . . heavier work for able-bodied men . . . cleaning the compound . . . cooking . . . one man doing carpentry work, asking for more tools to train younger men and boys . . . ward-servants . . . a new fence to keep out cattle . . . the women are overjoyed with a loom . . . goats are kept by some individuals . . . cows have been promised.' Moulmein was busy, happy, cheerful and largely untouched by the war-stories which reached it from Europe and China.

But Burma, like the whole of Europe, was soon to be a battlefield. The hospitals would be over-run, the patients dispersed, those of the staff who did not escape interned. No part of the Mission's work would be unaffected by the war.

13: Two Victorian Ladies

While Father Damien caught the imagination of the whole world, The Mission to Lepers had its own heroines – two Victorian ladies. Mary Reed was an American missionary and Rosalie Harvey went to India from England. They both lived out their lives there, though they never met, and remained truly Victorian until their deaths at the time of World War II.

Mary Reed was born in Ohio, USA, a few years before Wellesley Bailey first crossed the road to visit the beggars in Ambala. In 1884 she was accepted as a Methodist missionary to women in India and the following year began her work in Cawnpore. In the hot weather she fell ill and was sent up to the hills to recuperate and begin her language study at Pithoragarh. She was shocked to be told there were five hundred men, women and children in the district who suffered from leprosy, and even more distressed when she saw them.

Five years later, on her first leave in the USA, she felt a constant tingling sensation in her finger and noticed a patch under one ear. Without telling her family she consulted her own doctor and then went to see specialists who confirmed what she suspected. Without confiding in anyone but her sister, she returned to India knowing that she had leprosy, and equally certain that God had given her leprosy for his own purposes. Those purposes were that she should give her whole life to his children in the Indian hills who also suffered from leprosy! Her decision to go back to the Himalayas was as dramatic in its way as Father Damien's sudden offer, in the middle of a church service, to go to Molokai.

The American Methodists had no budget for her to do leprosy work but when The Mission to Lepers was approached for help Wellesley Bailey agreed and she became the only direct missionary appointment on the Mission's books for thirty years. Bailey appointed her superintendent of the Mission at Chandag, a lovely, remote place some 6,500 feet up in the Himalayan foothills.

In time her disease appeared to go into remission and in later years she showed no signs of leprosy at all, but she never attempted or even wanted to leave Chandag and her friends amongst the hill-people. Especially she never doubted or resented the call that sent her to them.

Within a year or two she had sixty-four leprosy patients, of whom forty-nine had become Christians, and the numbers grew year by year. With their help she built a small house for herself, a guest house for visitors, and building after building for the leprosy sufferers themselves. Criticised by villagers for allowing her patients to 'pollute' the drinking water she trudged the hills until she found a spring which could be piped to her own compound. Schools were opened in Chandag and in the nearby hill-villages and, after training village girls to teach in them, she tramped through the hills to maintain contact with teachers and schools and to preach.

The long dress with its narrow waist and bustle in which she arrived in the 1880s eventually gave place to long skirts, white blouses and an immense sun-topi – and that style of dress she maintained until her frail old age. There were other things that remained the same, too. The simplicity of her faith and the love she gave to her patients went on unchanged; so did the welcome she gave to visitors who penetrated the hills and valley to come to Chandag.

Though the American press headlined her story and then forgot about her, to children in Sunday school and to supporters of The Mission to Lepers the story of 'the missionary who had leprosy' was for fifty years a sharply-focused reminder that leprosy must not be forgotten. If

Mary Reed could give so much, how could other people withhold their support?

Rosalie Harvey was a very different kind of woman in a very different setting.

She was born at Seaford, in Sussex, England, in 1884 into a vicar's family and it was no surprise when she offered for service in India with the Zenana Bible and Medical Mission. In 1882 she landed in Bombay, fell ill and nearly died soon afterwards, and was sent to Poona to recuperate. Then, in 1884, she was stationed at Nasik, a 'holy city' with thousands of Hindu pilgrims.

Rosalie Harvey was interested in the temples and their worship because, like another famous Indian missionary, Amy Carmichael of Dohnavur, she was appalled that deserted or unwanted children were sold to the temples for the service of the gods and, whether they were boys or girls, became religious prostitutes. Like Amy Carmichael she set out to rescue at least some of the children and provide them with a home.

The compound of her house, however, held not only a great many boys and girls but a host of animals, too – sick buffaloes, worn-out bullocks, donkeys with broken legs, wounded dogs . . . all of them welcomed by this woman who could not pass any living thing in need or distress. Throughout the Nasik area she was a familiar, if slightly bizarre, figure for though the Victorian age gave way to different fashions Rosalie Harvey never changed her own – a long black skirt, white blouse, tight black cap over scraped-back hair with its little bun, blonde at first and then going grey.

The Indians had their own name for her, coined out of love – and out of her own love for everyone in need.

'*Aayi!*' they saluted her whenever they saw her – 'Mother!' After only a few years she was known everywhere by that name. Tireless in her service, she was relentless in her determination to have justice for those in need, whether they were sick animals, unwanted children . . . or sufferers from leprosy.

She had been in Nasik for fourteen years before famine ravaged the whole of eastern India, and that was followed by plague. The people who suffered most in Nasik were the beggars, all of them with leprosy, who made the verandah of the Naru Shanker temple their home. If no one gave them charity the beggars would starve. Rosalie Harvey pleaded their cause with the municipal authorities and gained them a daily food ration and, when the emergency had passed, begged money to build them a shelter. A Parsee businessman gave her 175 rupees – just enough to buy fourteen sheets of corrugated iron and construct a metal shed for some of the sufferers. By 1903 there was a permanent leprosy home. *Aayi* had committed herself to yet another kind of despised family.

When her first appeal for help arrived Wellesley Bailey had already told his Committee that there were no more funds however deserving the cause. That was when the new magazine, *Without the Camp*, first proved its value in publicity and fund-raising, running a special appeal for her work.

From the appearance of that first article *Aayi*'s story caught the imagination. There were more and more buildings, more and more leprosy sufferers given help. The quality of her work was recognised by the government of India who gave her their highest award for public service, the Kaiser-i-Hind Gold Medal – though she refused to come and receive it in public from the Governor of the Province for she coveted no rewards and no public applause. All she asked was the time, the energy and the support to serve her friends, the men, women and children who had leprosy and to whom she could give nothing but love.

14: A World at War

1939: September	– Germany invaded Poland and Britain and France declared war.
1940: April/May	– Germany overran Denmark, Norway, Holland and Belgium.
June	– France capitulated and British forces were evacuated from Dunkirk.
1940/41	– British cities 'blitzed'.
1941: December	– Japan attacked American fleet in Pearl Harbour, Honolulu.
1942: Spring	– Japan occupied the Philippines, South East Asia, Burma and Indonesia.
1943: Autumn	– Allies invaded Italy from North Africa; Italy capitulated but war continued in Europe and Asia.
1945: May	– Germany surrendered.
1945: August	– Japan surrendered, after atomic bombs had been dropped on Hiroshima and Nagasaki.

Only those who lived through them know the pressures and tragedies hidden behind that summary of six years of anguish. At the Mission's headquarters the staff shared all the problems of those who lived or worked in London. Travel was difficult; homes were bombed; local meetings were curtailed by the blackout; news from Asia was increasingly scarce and, as the Japanese consolidated their gains, ceased altogether from China and Burma. It was no surprise when William Anderson announced that he wished to retire at the end of 1942. He had given outstanding leadership, initiated important changes of policy and had had the joy of seeing 'the new treatment' providing vigour and health where for so long there had been only despair.

It was agreed that Donald Miller, the Secretary for India, should return to London and take his place as General Secretary, while Wilfrid Russell in Faizabad took over in India. Mr and Mrs Miller had an intimate knowledge of the Mission's work throughout India – and amongst Mrs Miller's 'mementos' was a compass she had used in Purulia. It was, before long, to save their lives.

While change was being planned in London more shattering upheavals were taking place in Asia. When war broke out in the west the Japanese already had a stranglehold on China. Foreigners, including missionaries, were interned and as leprosy work in China had been maintained by foreign missions, including The Mission to Lepers, leprosy hospitals and homes virtually came to an end. Even after Pearl Harbour, however, Europeans in Asia saw little reason for panic for a time, persuaded of the impregnable defences in Singapore and the Dutch strength in the East Indies. Their confidence was disastrously shattered. Java and Sumatra were overrun and Singapore capitulated in February, 1942. At Easter, four months after Japan had entered the war, Mandalay was bombed and its teak houses set on fire. Moulmein had already been occupied. Clem Chapman, the Methodist minister who had oversight of the Mandalay leprosy home, led a shocked congregation in Easter worship amongst the smouldering ruins of the church, and then set off with a group of refugees northwards through the teak forests. He reached Assam alone, exhausted and in rags, with only his dog for companion. Leprosy work in Burma ended and the patients dispersed; and even in Assam it ceased for some time.

When Donald Miller and his wife left India in the autumn of 1942 Burma was already lost, the Japanese threatened to break through the Assam defences and to overrun Bengal – and the sea-lanes between Asia, Africa and

Europe were far from safe. The Millers reached Cape Town and continued their journey in the steamship *City of Cairo*. Six days later, on 6th November, while they were at dinner there was a shuddering crash below the water-line and the lights went out. The ship had been torpedoed. There was no panic, no shouting; but equally no time to go to cabins for coats or the ready-packed bags of treasured possessions. From the six lifeboats which had been successfully launched those who had escaped watched as the submarine surfaced to make sure the ship sank – as it did only twenty-three minutes after it was hit.

When morning came the Millers found themselves with fifty-five people in the twenty-eight-foot lifeboat. They had little precise knowledge of where they were, or which direction to steer – and when the compass was taken out of the locker it had been splintered in the explosion. It was then that Mrs Miller took her treasure from her coat pocket.

'I've got a compass here! It's the one I used with Guides at the leprosy hospital at Purulia!'

With it they made a safe but slow way across the ocean until, after thirteen days, they were picked up by a cargo vessel bound for Glasgow.

They landed in Britain with only the clothes they wore; with an experience of what it meant to be almost without hope; but thankful that they were alive. Donald Miller could now take over from William Anderson. William Anderson, however, was dead. He had collapsed in the street just after Christmas, 1942, on his way to meet members of the Mission's Council in the City of London. Miller was left to pick up the reins of office without the friendly guidance of a great Secretary who had given forty years of his life to the leprosy sufferers of Asia.

Anderson had taken over towards the end of one war and Miller took over in the middle of another, but there were vast differences in their inheritances. Not only in the size of the budget and the number of patients being cared for but in the attitude to leprosy itself. Though the new chaulmoogra treatment was not the universal cure that had first been hoped it was widely recognised that some forms of leprosy could be cured and patients were being discharged symptom-free – and, at least as important, many of them were being accepted back into community life, even though the old terrors of leprosy had by no means completely disappeared. A letter from Stanley Jones, the missionary at Raniganj in Bengal, exemplified some of the new attitudes.

'Monilal, one of our Scouts and an outside-left in our football team, was discharged as symptom-free and is now in charge of a group of labourers at one of the aerodromes ... Radha Gopal is making splendid progress at high school and was second in the annual exams ... Kulabala Sircar is about to take her finals as a nurse in Jaigung hospital ... Lekjhan Mundal came to see us and told us how well she is doing in the weaving school.'

From Africa, however, came indications that the scene was changing even more swiftly and dramatically.

At Uzuakoli in Nigeria Dr James Kinnear Brown had once founded an agricultural settlement for leprosy sufferers expelled from Port Harcourt and abandoned on territory believed to be cursed by the medicine men. In 1939 Brown was joined by Dr Frank Davey, a doctor and minister of the Methodist Missionary Society who was to rank with such pioneers as Dr Stanley Browne and Dr Paul Brand. Under the leadership of a maimed but greatly gifted leprosy sufferer, Harcourt White, Frank Davey gathered some 800 patients into mud-huts – and saw the beginnings of the great Uzuakoli Leprosy Settlement. Unhappily largely destroyed in the Nigerian civil war it is now recreated and active once more.

Davey was then joined by Dr John Lowe, a biochemist who had worked in the Tropical Medicine School in Calcutta and was a close associate of Dr Ernest Muir, so much linked with The Mission to Lepers. Few people knew what was happening in Uzuakoli, and even fewer were aware that it was one of the places chosen for experiment with yet another new drug. A letter from Frank Davey, in 1942, made astonishing reading.

'The work of the Colony grows apace. We now have more than 6,000 patients and are supervising no fewer than twenty-nine out-station clinics. *This year I shall be discharging at least 150 as symptom-free and if staff permitted the work could be extended indefinitely* ... 5,000 of the patients are from this area but there are probably another 10,000 who are not in our care. The figures are staggering but we are not dismayed, and you are giving us great assistance.'

The statistics *were* staggering. But the deeper interest lay in the remarkable discoveries that made it possible to discharge so many as symptom-free so quickly.

The doctors at Uzuakoli were no longer using the 'new treatment' with chaulmoogra oil. They had moved forward to yet another treatment and they were not alone in their experiments. In the United States and other parts of the world leprologists and research centres were at work developing and testing – and, if the results at Uzuakoli were a true indication of what could happen, perhaps offering to the world, at last, the answer they had so long been seeking.

15: The Fight Against Leprosy: DDS (1935–1950s)

The DDS episode is probably the most involved, and perhaps the most fascinating, story in the whole history of the struggle with leprosy.

Behind it is the fact the most effective weapon had been put aside on the shelves of a German chemist in 1908.

There were, in fact, three men concerned in the scientific work of that apparently unimportant affair. Fromm and Whitman were working on water pollution and Gelmo on another project. Both groups discovered compounds of sulphone, but these were not relevant to their immediate needs. The drug was shelved. It could not have occurred to any of them that it might one day have any significance in the leprosy situation.

Only in 1935 did it emerge again when another German chemist, Gerhardt Domack, produced a drug for a chemical firm which was patented under the name of prontosil. It earned its discoverer a Nobel prize because it was shown to destroy bacteria which caused many deadly diseases, but other scientists – and drug firms, too – disliked the limitations imposed on its use by its having being patented. In several countries there was research to try and 'beat the ban' and discover the chemical structure of prontosil. In France four scientists at the Pasteur Institute eventually found that the active element in prontosil was amino-benzine-sulphonamide. It was the same element which Gelmo had synthesised and abandoned on his shelves in 1908! One result was the possibility of manufacturing sulphonamide, and from this came the production of various remedies, the best known to the general public being the mysterious-sounding M & B 693.

Researchers at the Pasteur Institute and a group at the Wellcome Institute in London under Dr Buttle continued to investigate the sulphones which until then had been largely neglected. When Dr Buttle accidentally discovered the sulphones he was, in fact, investigating the action of sulphonamides in combating typhoid and pneumonia. It was then that one of his chemists – to quote a scientific writer about what occurred – 'happened to come across' diamino-diphenyl-sulphone. As 'DDS' it was to move into the world of leprosy with quite staggering impact, although at that time no one associated DDS – or dapsone, as it came to be called – with that disease. There was a very good reason why they did not. The newer chemists found the same thing which Gelmo had found in 1908 – the drug was too toxic for use with human beings. *It would poison those who were treated with it!*

The story, in another of its convolutions, then moved across the Atlantic. A chemist named Tillotson, working for Parke Davis and Co in Detroit, produced a far less toxic form of the drug which he named Promin.

It was at that point that leprosy came into the story for the first time. But, in order to understand how it did so, it is necessary to go back to the days following the American Civil War.

After that conflict was over and the slaves were legally emancipated throughout America, while southern gentry looked across impoverished estates at rows of empty slave-huts, New Orleans had become one of the roughest and most uninhibited towns in the Southern states. Criminals, thieves and prostitutes were everywhere. But there was one place which even they shunned – Dr Beard's Pest House with its frightening inhabitants, all of them sufferers from leprosy. It was not until 1894 that the authorities decided, for the peace of mind of the rest of the city, that they should be moved away down-river to an old, decaying mansion, the Indian Camp Plantation near the village of Carville. The workers lived in the mansion, the leprosy patients in the empty slave cabins, segregated from the rest of the world by high wire fences, and males from females in the same way. Two years later four nuns arrived from the Daughters of the Sisters of Charity of St Vincent de Paul, and gave the sufferers rather more loving care.

Eventually, after decades of neglect and suffering, the run-down leprosy centre was taken over by the Federal government in 1921 and renamed, with a care to avoid the word 'leprosy', The United States Military Hospital, No 66. At this hospital Dr Guy Faget, who arrived in 1940, began experimental use of some of the sulphonamide drugs. Hearing of the new drug, promin, which had been produced by the Parke Davis company he wrote and enquired about it and was sent a supply of it.

Almost as soon as he attempted to treat patients with promin it was quite clear that something beyond his own – or anyone else's – experience had begun to happen. In this group of patients two were relieved of throat conditions that had needed operations, two were cleared of nasal infections, and one, nearly blind, was able to see. 'The Miracle at Carville' was headlined across the world, in medical journals as well as the popular press.

It was, however, far too expensive to consider treating the large numbers of leprosy sufferers in Asia and Africa with it. In Frank Davey's phrase it was 'heaven out of reach'.

Once more the story recrossed the Atlantic, to Britain.

In 1945 Dr Robert Cochrane touched down by seaplane in Poole Harbour, Dorset. He was Principal of the Christian Medical College in Vellore, South India, deeply involved with The Mission to Lepers, and had come to undertake a fund-raising tour through Britain and Ireland on the Mission's behalf. Most congregations in this immediate post-war period were, however, much more concerned about rebuilding in Britain following war damage than about leprosy sufferers in

India. Cochrane had an unrewarding tour until he reached Belfast. Even then what rewarded him was not money or the promise of it but a conversation over a coffee-table!

Cochrane had been speaking about the new DDS derivatives, and touched on the frustration that leprosy workers were feeling because these were financially inaccessible. A professor, over coffee, mentioned that an agricultural scientist in Cheshire had been injecting pure DDS, not its derivatives such as promin, into the udders of cows to counteract mastitis. Cochrane immediately developed a hunch that there could be a link between the successful treatment of the Cheshire cows, and a treatment for leprosy patients, and when he returned to India he took with him a supply of DDS.

There were doubts and failures before success came – but it did come. By using small doses of DDS – far less expensive than the derivatives which demanded many more processes – and giving it by mouth instead of by injections a remarkable change began to take place amongst patients.

Cochrane in India and Davey in Nigeria were two of the people around the world pioneering the reduction of DDS to an acceptable dosage and, in doing so, reducing the cost of treatment. Work in other parts of the world confirmed their findings. From workers in Brazil, Malaya and Guyana came the same kind of information.

Dapsone would not, by itself, be able to eradicate leprosy from the world but it was a far more effective weapon than anything previously discovered. It would, as time would quickly show, provide treatment for the less virulent form of leprosy and send patients home symptom-free far more quickly than ever before.

But, from the standpoint of The Mission to Lepers, this newest treatment would involve them, and all the bigger hospitals whether they were run by missions, church or state, in an entirely different way of life.

16: Now That the War Was Over (1945–60)

Now that the war was over towns and cities would need rebuilding, in Britain and on the continent of Europe. In Britain rationing remained in force; essential supplies were limited; the old workhouses for the indigent poor were still in existence. Needs at the other end of the world seemed even further away than in pre-war days. In this traumatic climate of change, however, not everything took a turn for the worse. In the World Health Organization there was a reaction against the use of the word leper and it was banned by the WHO within a few years after the war. The American Mission to Lepers followed the lead of WHO and rejected it as a degrading word, although it was twenty years before the title of The Mission to Lepers was changed in Britain – and even then there would be supporters who felt that much of the emotional impact was lost!

Donald Miller remained the General Secretary, though Wilfrid Russell was brought from India in 1953 to assist him in his ever-growing responsibilities, and throughout this period some of the most significant developments in the history of the Mission took place, with hints of greater changes yet to come. They included the new drugs; a changing policy about Mission appointments; a completely fresh element in leprosy treatment – orthopaedic surgery; a changed attitude to the high cost of research; a notable increase in income; and both advance and withdrawals overseas.

The new sulphone drugs provided far more dramatic results than the chaulmoogra injections, with their pain and frequent side-effects. Pills were much easier to take, and even lepromatous patients, who for years had been resigned to eventually dying in hospital, began to have a measure of new hope. Doctors who shunned a phrase like 'miracle drug' nevertheless discharged patients as symptom-free for whom they had had little hope. And patients themselves, going back to the world outside, had no inhibitions in telling everyone that they were 'cured'.

On Miller's first-ever tour of Africa he came to Itu, a great leprosy colony in Nigeria managed by Church of Scotland missionaries. There were 2000 patients in the colony and all of them, that day, crowded into the huge church. Some hobbled on broken feet; some could hardly do more than crawl; others were blind. But there were those who walked upright and pushed toward the front where the superintendent stood with a paper in his hand. What followed took a long time – though time had mattered little in a leprosy colony where most patients had expected to spend the rest of their lives. The superintendent read out names, 286 in all, and after each name came shouts of joy from all the congregation. The service which followed was typically African – uninhibited rejoicing and praise to God who healed and gave new life.

This was a typical 'Discharge Announcement Ceremony' in the great African leprosy colonies. Nearly three hundred people were able to return to the villages which had once forced them away.

Only a year or so after the introduction of sulphone drugs the American Leprosy Mission sent half a million DDS tablets to their British counterpart for use in India. Soon they were being used throughout the world. The number of patients discharged grew year by year and four dramatic, almost incredible, words of hope reverberated across the world.

'Leprosy *can* be cured!'

By the 1960s and '70s wards full of long-term residents were to give place to busy out-patient departments – for the first time, the fight against leprosy was being carried from the hospital into the village, the countryside and the bush.

In the post-war world of new nations which began with Indian independence in 1947, missionary societies faced conditions very different from the pre-war imperial world. New native churches or conferences took over from western-based missionary societies, usually with the warm encouragement of the old societies. From both sides there was a strong desire that relationships should be unimpaired and missionaries would be available as fully as the new national churches wished. But it was not quite as easy as that, not merely because white Christians did not feel as urgent a call to serve overseas, but also because new independent governments, for many reasons, were unwilling to allow foreigners back in their pre-war numbers unless they had knowledge or skills which their own nationals did not possess. One result was that there were fewer missionaries whom the societies could send to leprosy work. In turn The Mission to Lepers, which had relied so much on doctors, nurses and ancillary workers belonging to other missions, now had to appoint an increasing number of its own missionaries. Leprosy workers were generally welcome in the new nations because this was an area in which not enough nationals had the necessary expertise.

In the early 1950s a new name began to feature in reports from India. Paul Brand was born in India of missionary parents, had trained in Britain in orthopaedic surgery and, back in India, went for a time to the great Christian hospital at Vellore. But the work to which he committed himself would involve much experiment and research and there were those who felt that this was not the proper task of The Mission to Lepers. Dr Muir, one of the most respected Christian leprologists, had warned the Mission's Council in 1948 that: 'Research is not our business. It would cost too much money!'

However, when it came to research the Americans had no such hesitations. As early as 1946 the American Mission had offered a large grant for the establishment of research work at Vellore though it was not until 1953 that the sanatorium for adult patients was opened at Karigiri, some miles from Vellore. By this time The Mission to Lepers had shared the building costs equally with the American mission. It was to be known as the Schieffelin Leprosy Research Institute in honour of the first President of the American Mission to Lepers who had begun his association with that work in 1906. Two years after it was opened he died, but the institute that carried his name was to become one of the leprosy world's greatest training-centres, including orthopaedic surgery with its restoration of hands and feet. Trainees would be welcomed and go back enriched from Asia, Africa, the Pacific and the West.

It had also been proposed to build a children's sanatorium at Vellore but in the end that was opened at Faizabad, Wellesley Bailey's first home in India.

On Donald Miller's post-war overseas tours he found encouragement in some places and sadness in others. There were, in 1948, some 10,000 patients in homes owned or aided by the Mission, and in India, where the new government was concerned about leprosy work, new buildings and extensions were going up steadily. Perhaps the most touching story was from the Himalayan foothills. There the courageous American woman, Mary Reed, who had served the leprosy sufferers of the hills until she died a year or so after the war began, would have rejoiced (however humbly) at the Memorial Hospital bearing her name which replaced the old wooden house in which she had lived.

In India leprosy work had not greatly suffered from World War II, but in Burma the patients had fled from the homes as soon as Japanese forces began to overrun the country. Now, as the Japanese retreated and finally surrendered, they came back to bombed churches and empty buildings with neither doctors nor Christian workers to welcome them. Wearing rags, or coverings made from the gunny-bags in which the Japanese soldiers kept their provisions, they were a sad sight with sores and ulcers. Because they had suffered so much from malnutrition, even when help reached them many of them inevitably died.

At least in Burma, however, it was possible to plan for the future. In China that was not the case. Under Chairman Mao's government relationships with Christian churches in the West and in America were severed and were not restored for many years. For the links which were established by the mission in the 1950s were not with mainland China but the colony of Hong Kong – a remarkable story which will be told in chapter twenty-four.

In 1955 yet another war assaulted eastern Asia – the Korean war which left the north and south of that country completely divided. In the south the continuance of some splendid leprosy work was guaranteed.

This chapter would seem to imply that Asia dominated the Mission's plans, reports and budgets – and until the 1950s this was largely true. It had done so for eighty years, since the beginning. But after Miller made an extensive secretarial tour of Africa that continent was to figure much more often. One reason that contributed to the new 'African interest' was that in the Belgian Congo, at a remote bush station called Yalisambo, the Millers met and heard remarkable stories from a very remarkable man – an English doctor named Stanley Browne. His story will be told in chapter twenty-nine. Together with Paul Brand he provided pioneering initiatives which helped to transform the whole of leprosy work.

17: The Fight Against Leprosy: New Hands for Old (1945 onwards)

Paul Brand was born, in 1914, to strict Baptist missionary parents in south India and sent to England with his sister for schooling in London. Ill-disciplined and daringly adventurous he nevertheless had a youthful dedication which deepened into a driving commitment to Christ and his purpose. Part of that purpose Paul saw as being a missionary like his unconventional father and, like him, he did a year's simple medical training at the Livingstone Medical School. He then went on to study medicine at University College, London, where he married a fellow-student, Margaret Berry, and urged on by her doctor father, gained his FRCS.

In 1946 came an astonishing telegram. '. . . urgent need for surgeon to teach at Vellore . . . come immediately on short-term contract.' It was signed 'Cochrane' and Paul could not believe it.

Vellore was the great Christian medical college in South India, now being up-graded to meet the high demands of the Indian government. Robert Cochrane, brilliant, forceful and determined, had been seconded to Vellore for this transitional period to see it properly established in its new role, though he retained his post as Superintendent of the nearby Chingleput Leprosy Hospital – a government institution, staffed by the Church and supported by The Mission to Lepers. But Vellore had only one surgeon, an

American Baptist, and a second was needed. Cochrane believed Paul Brand was the man he wanted – and, leaving Margaret and the baby to join him in a year's time, Paul set off for Vellore.

Back 'home' in south India Paul plunged with immense enthusiasm into his surgical and teaching work, surrounded by students who copied his mannerisms almost as eagerly as they did his techniques.

He had been there some time before Dr Cochrane invited him to take time off and visit Chingleput.

'I'd be glad to do that,' he replied. 'I haven't really seen lepers at close quarters.'

Cochrane's response was explosive. 'We don't have *lepers* at Chingleput. It's a *leprosy* hospital and we have *patients who suffer from leprosy*. Don't use that word! It's offensive!'

Much chastened, Paul walked through the Chingleput hospital compound and was shattered by what he saw in those pre-sulphone days. People with ulcerated feet, some semi-blind, others with noses that had become flattened – but one thing above all others horrified this young surgeon – people's *hands*. Their fingers were 'clawed', bent inwards stiffly and apparently almost useless.

'Why don't you *do* something about hands like these?', he demanded.

Cochrane swung round on him. 'Why do *you* ask *me*? I'm not an orthopaedic surgeon! *You* are! Do you know that there are millions of people with leprosy in the world – and I don't believe one single orthopaedic surgeon has ever done any work on leprosy!'

Brand felt as if he had been hit in the face. 'Let me see your hands', he said to a young man. They were thrust out obediently, fingers tightly bent inwards, useless for gripping anything. 'Take hold of my hand', Brand said. He slid his hand between the clawed fingers – and winced sharply, drawing it out and massaging it. 'That hand *isn't* useless! There are muscles that still work'. He could still feel the vice-like grip of the man's 'useless' hand. 'Perhaps they *all* have muscles that would work if we could find a way of re-shaping them?'

The young surgeon's visit to Chingleput must rank with Wellesley Bailey's crossing the road to sit with the leprosy sufferers of Ambala nearly a century earlier. It marked the beginning of a completely new phase in leprosy work.

Because he was employed as surgeon and teacher at Vellore any research work had to be fitted into spare hours but the young professor managed to enthuse some of his colleagues, especially a Sinhalese woman doctor, Gusta Buultgens. She shared a postmortem examination of a beggar who had had leprosy, and whose hands were literally taken to pieces by the light of an oil lamp. It must have been reminiscent of Armauer Hansen's postmortems at Bergen in the earliest days of the discovery of the leprosy bacillus. This beggar, too, contributed more in death than he had ever done in life. There *were* working muscles. Surely, felt Brand, and his Sinhalese colleague, it should be possible to transplant tendons into fingers and thumbs, tie them in with working muscles in the arms – and provide leprosy patients with hands that would 'work' again?

The theory turned into living fact in 1948. A well-educated young man named Krishnamurty, who had been turned out to beg when it was discovered that he had leprosy, made a compliant but unenthusiastic 'guinea pig'. He had nothing to lose and did not believe he had anything to gain. Let the British doctor do what he wanted! There was a long series of meticulous operations, exposing tendons, splitting them, layering them into fingers, knotting them in with working muscles, massaging and exercising and flexing unused fingers ... and at last Krishnamurty had two, then three, then four fingers on each hand – fingers that worked!

Between them, surgeon and patient had proved that leprosy sufferers could have new hands for old.

By the time he left hospital Krishnamurty had not only new hands but a new name. He had come to see Jesus as the source of life and had been baptised as 'John'.

Brand's colleagues were fascinated though some were only half-convinced. What about the 'bad flesh' of leprosy sufferers? It was generally accepted that fingers 'fell off', and they were certainly very often shortened. Brand persuaded colleagues to examine flesh from living patients in many places over long periods. The answer was always the same. Surprisingly so. 'This flesh is as normal as anyone else's!' There wasn't any 'bad flesh'. So why did fingers fall off, bit by bit?

The next step in finding an answer came when Brand saw a boy with a clawed hand turning a key in a lock. The task was difficult but the boy, with his hands long anaesthetised as leprosy destroyed the nerves under the skin-surface, had no feeling of how hard the key cut into his hands, and he took no notice when the blood dripped from the frayed skin on his fingers. Brand had already seen leprosy patients pick up hot pots from the fire without knowing that the deadened hands were burned down to the bone. They did not even notice the smell of burning flesh.

Such injuries produced the ulcers that needed constant treatment – but for the first time it was realised that these injuries were the reason why fingers seemed to be shortened and 'drop off'. There was no 'bad flesh'. It was worn away by accident or misuse or burned away from the anaesthetised fingers. Elementary though the answer proved to be it had taken a century to show that 'bad flesh' was false doctrine – and there were doctors closely in touch with leprosy work who for years still refused to believe it.

It was a few months after his first patient had been discharged that John came back to Vellore hospital. 'These hands are no good', he complained.

They examined them and found the fingers worked, and that nothing was wrong.

'No', explained John. 'I don't mean that. They are no good for begging! When I sit in the bazaar with a begging-bowl people look at my hands and give me nothing.'

So 'new hands' did not mean 'new life'! Leprosy sufferers, cured and discharged, could not find work. Fortunately John had once been able to type and with his newly-flexible fingers he was able to do so again. Even if people did not all have skills of that kind they could surely, if given the chance, develop *some* ability to work? With a generous gift from an eighty-four-year-old American woman missionary, 'Mother' Eaton, a new village was created on part of the Vellore Hospital site – Nava Jeeva Nilayan, the 'New Life Centre'. Not intended as a permanent refuge it was a preparation for the future; a collection of small, simple huts like those to which the villagers would return, a place in which leprosy-sufferers now symptom-free, with useable hands, could learn a trade they could follow in the world outside instead of having to beg for a living.

This in itself, of course, was not enough. Hands with new tendons, fingers that moved, were by no means effective instruments for office work or even manual skills. There was need for carefully-adapted physiotherapy, for months or perhaps longer. Ruth Thomas, a missionary working in Hong Kong, came to Vellore as its first highly competent physiotherapist. Nava Jeeva Nilayan was a triumphant success-story. Dr Hilda Lazarus, Principal of the College, took great interest in it and helped to develop its atmosphere of beauty and hope. By 1954 it had its own operating-theatre. Medical students moving freely between college, hospital and village began a new attitude, breaking down their inherent antipathy to those who had leprosy. Some, in time, would help to spread the news not only that leprosy could be cured but that leprosy need not be feared.

Both Paul and Margaret Brand took other very important steps forward in these years. Dr Margaret Brand moved into eye-surgery and contributed greatly in an area so far untouched in the rehabilitation of leprosy sufferers. And, as he had done with hands, Paul Brand moved on to adapt his hand-surgery techniques to feet, and offer 'new feet for old', too. The inherent problem that followed this successful operation was to find the right sort of shoes for long-damaged, still mis-shapen and often unfeeling feet. It was a long and often disappointing quest with success long-delayed.

Within ten years of going to Vellore Paul Brand was known throughout the world as an outstanding contributor to leprosy work. By 1959, when over 5,000 hand-operations had been successfully carried out, trainees and specialists from every continent had begun coming to Karigiri, the training centre near Vellore, and going back with fresh techniques and new hopes, including the place of physiotherapy in the process of rehabilitation.

But Dr Paul Brand was not permitted to remain in south India as a highly able Christian surgeon in a Christian hospital. In 1965 he was persuaded to take up an appointment at Carville, Louisiana, USA – the place which had once been a dilapidated southern mansion taken over to house leprosy sufferers in the unused slave-huts. It had gone on to be a military hospital for soldiers with the then-feared disease, and was greatly involved in the development of the DDS story. It was to be Paul Brand's base for many years and it was from here that he was called to visit every part of the world. One example of his wider commitment to the service of leprosy sufferers was the part he played in the setting up of the major African research and training centre, ALERT, in Addis Ababa. He would continue to be closely associated with The Leprosy Mission, but his contribution would be world-wide, over-leaping national and church dividing-lines.

18: The Fight Against Leprosy: The Emptying Wards (1950s onwards)

By the 1950s DDS tablets were as cheap as aspirins and were in use throughout the world. There were two notable results.

The first, which gave new heart to missionaries, national staff and patients, was that many sufferers who had been expected to spend many years in hospital were now going back to the world outside. Farewells, once rare, were becoming a normal feature of hospital life. 'Last evening,' wrote a missionary from West Africa, 'one hundred patients stood up at the Valedictory Service to hear the minister's words of farewell.' Another African comment was that '. . . there aren't enough "well" patients left in the wards to help look after the sick ones!'

The other result, within the hospitals themselves, was a sense of hope that transformed drudgery and tedium into vigour and excitement. U Ba Aye, later to become President of the Burmese Methodist Conference, described the feelings at Mandalay—where he was manager of the leprosy home—'Groups of women are helping with the weaving which supplies all our needs of bandages and gauze, and also teaching the girls how to weave. Groups help in turn with the cooking for the hospitalised patients and the ulcer wards. Masons and carpenters help in the building and repair programme, and a number of male and female patients help in the wards.' The significant word, repeated in this and other letters, is 'help'. Hope produced a new readiness to share in the world of healing.

This, indeed, was said quite explicitly in a letter from Faizabad. 'What was once "just another job to do" is rapidly becoming "a task worth doing well". More and more often you see the smile that says: "*I* had a part in helping this man to get better!"'

Nor was it only bodies which were healed. Morning and evening prayers, ward services, testimonies in outpatients departments and personal witness to Christ by patients and staff meant that the source of Christian compassion was made very clear. There were always some patients who were changed in heart as well as healed in body before they went home. The Mission to Lepers was not a proselytising agency, dealing with bodies in the hope of gaining souls – and that must always be underlined – but those who served it loved Jesus and wanted to share his love for them and for others. That was why they were where they were. 'The main object of the Mission', says the Constitution, 'is to minister in the name of Jesus Christ to the physical, mental and spiritual needs of sufferers from leprosy, to assist in their rehabilitation and to work towards the eradication of leprosy.' The love of Jesus was shared by loving ministry as much as by word.

Wards were becoming emptier not only because people were being discharged but because they were not replaced by long-term patients. The focus of the leprosy hospital's work had shifted. *It was no longer inside the walls, but outside.* 'In-patients' were giving way to 'out-patients'. Naturally sufferers needing constant observation or under special treatment or with some ancillary disease had to be in the wards, but if leprosy sufferers could be kept under observation in out-patients's clinics at the hospital or near their own home, or if treatment consisted of dapsone pills, there was no need for them to come into hospital at all. What at first seemed like a revolutionary approach to the world's most feared disease was very quickly accepted as normal. People who would have hidden the signs of their disease for as long as possible were now more ready to come for help, often

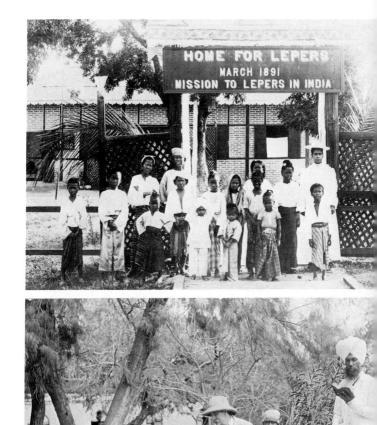

Top: The new home at Mandalay. *Bottom:* Literacy lessons for leprosy patients at Tarn Taran.

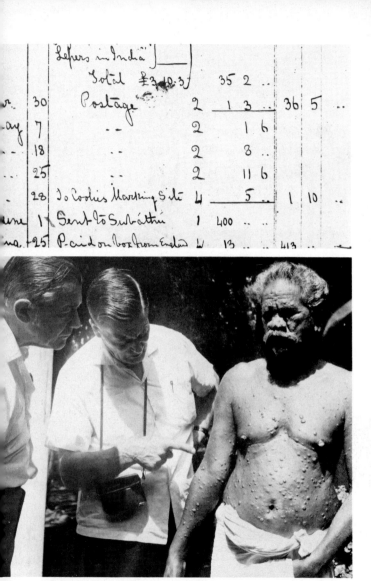

Top: An extract from Wellesley Bailey's cash book for 1875.
Bottom: Dr Paul Brand and Dr Stanley Browne sharing their expertise at Karigiri.

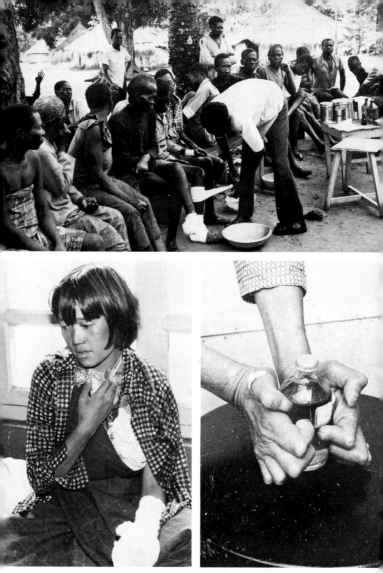

Top: Most people with leprosy are treated at out-patient clinics.
Bottom left: After surgery at Gida Kom, Bhutan.
Bottom right: 'Clawed' hands find it hard to perform the tasks we take for granted.

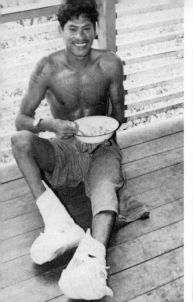

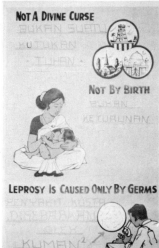

NOT A DIVINE CURSE

NOT BY BIRTH

LEPROSY IS CAUSED ONLY BY GERMS

KUMAN²

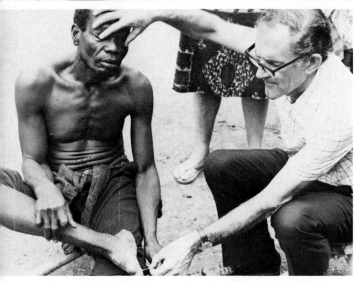

Top left: Damaged hands need not be a feature of leprosy.
Top right: Health education gradually breaks down prejudice against the disease. *Bottom:* Testing a patient for loss of feeling.

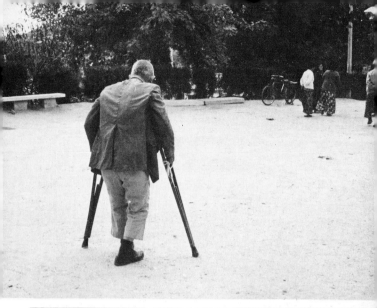

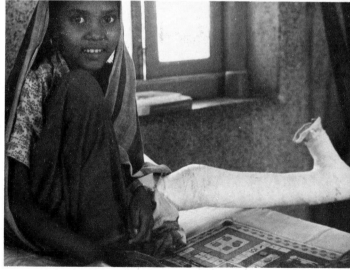

Top: Leprosy meant loneliness and disfigurement for an earlier generation. *Bottom:* Special care – and a game of Ludo – at Purulia, India.

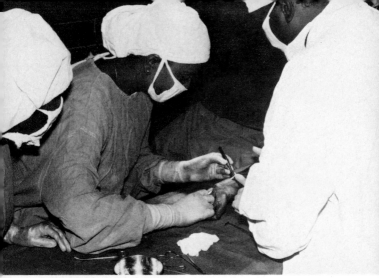

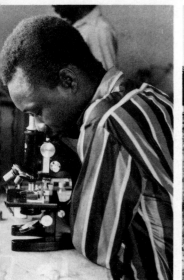

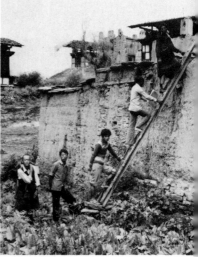

Top: Restoring movement to a damaged hand.
Bottom left: Laboratory technicians like Andrew are vital as part
of the back-up team in Zaire. *Bottom right:* In remote areas,
such as Bhutan, paramedics call at villagers' homes.

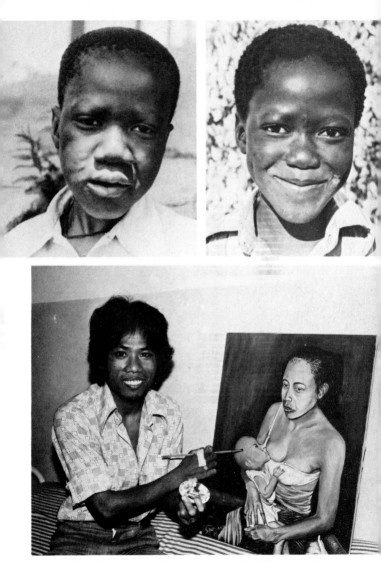

Top left: Pitso before he took treatment.... *Top right:* ...and one year later. *Bottom:* An excellent painter despite his deformed hands.

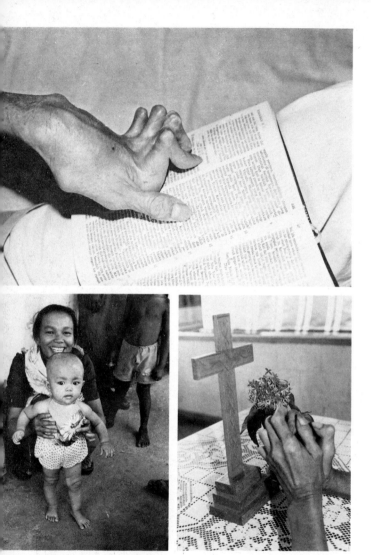

Top: Patients need much more than medicine.
Bottom left: Having taken treatment she won't pass the disease onto her child. *Bottom right:* The gospel is proclaimed in word and in action.

because the village 'grapevines' had passed the news from place to place that their situation was not as desperate as they had believed.

The reports which reached the Mission's headquarters in London reflected a completely new way of life.

Between Faizabad and Lucknow, in north India, was Barabanki. In 1961 the Faizabad hospital began an experimental 'country clinic' for villagers who would not travel the fifty miles or so to Faizabad. They thought that perhaps as many as a thousand people a year might take advantage of it. By the end of ten years over 40,000 people had received treatment in this out-patients clinic – and most of them had heard the gospel as well. At Karigiri, in south India, 2,000 patients came to the clinic in its first year and its work had to be limited to a twenty-mile radius to keep the number down to a compassable 4,000 a year. Africa, Korea, Thailand, or indeed the Himalayas and Papua New Guinea all provided stories of the same kind. But though the struggle was transferred from inside the hospital to the clinics outside, and though so many people took advantage of them, the most difficult problem still remained. That was that people, mostly in rural areas all over the world, who did not know that leprosy was curable would go on hiding their symptoms – and in some cases passing on the disease – as long as they could.

There were some long-term patients who could not be discharged into a hostile or unwelcoming world. Salakwanda Zulu was one of them. From the ward windows of Mbuluzi Leprosy Colony in Swaziland there was a splendid panorama of great stony hills beyond the deep valley below. Outside, the garden was bright with flowers. But Salakwanda could not see the flowers or the view. He had gone blind. Nor could he walk outside to feel the freshness of the air in the early morning, for he had no legs. Both conditions had arisen from his disease. How could such a man be 'the most cheerful patient in the home . . . the most radiant witness to the power of Christ'? The old, blind, legless man told everyone who would listen why he was so happy.

He was uneducated, shrewd and crooked in his younger days, smuggling drugs into Johannesburg, stealing when he could not get work, exultant in his wickedness – until he found he had leprosy. Driven out of Johannesburg by the police and out of his village in Swaziland by his own people, he existed with other sufferers like himself, hopeless and in deplorable squalour, until he heard Nazarene missionaries telling the story of Jesus and was converted. He found no relief for his leprosy but full forgiveness for his sins. Accepted for life at Mbuluzi he asked: 'How can I help being happy, even if I can't walk or see?'

In the sanctuary of the Christian hospital people like the one-time thief could find comfort and fellowship. But there were other sufferers, too, who could not join the out-patient queue.

Aisi was one of these people. She was born in a tiny village in Nepal. It was a hard life, like many other rural communities – especially for Aisi. She was married at twelve, according to custom, and then deserted by her husband who left her at her mother's house and never returned. Though they had scarcely enough to eat and Aisi's mother died, the real tragedy began when Aisi lost sensation in her hands and feet and developed ulceration. This could be nothing but leprosy, the curse of the gods. Two kindly neighbours escorted her on a long journey to Hardwar, the holy city in India, so that she could bathe in the sacred river Ganges, and wash away her sin. Once in Hardwar they left her in a *dharmasala*, a pilgrim-inn, and fled back to Nepal. Providentially she then met another leprosy-sufferer, an ex-patient from the Subathu hospital, so long supported by The Mission to Lepers, who offered to take her to the hospital. She was robbed of her small bundle on the train, containing her few clothes and her mother's precious silver bangles, and was quite prepared for the final disaster – to be rejected when she reached the hospital. Instead, as her 'testimony' ends, she was 'received with love – made rapid progress and recovered – and heard the name of the Saviour Jesus for the first time.'

There must always be a place for refugees like Aisi, wanderers with nowhere to go, who need love as much as they need healing.

Other reasons exist, too, for maintaining some kind of hospital 'base', whether it is a hospital like Vellore, a research-centre like Karigiri or a refugee-village and training centre like Shanti Nilayan. They indicate the contribution such places can make to full healing. 'New hands for old', and new feet, too, give the operating theatre and the surgical ward a new and special importance. Much of the early work of physiotherapy may need to be undertaken in a longer-term setting. The additional emphasis in the care of restored hands and feet which was developed after these first break-throughs was not only getting accustomed to *using* them but in particular training patients to *prevent* deformity and damage; even though fingers or feet were given new mobility they did not find *feeling* restored to them.

When Wilfrid Russell, who became General Secretary after Donald Miller retired, visited The Mission to Lepers' stations in the 1960s his mind must have raced back over his first years in North India in the 1930s. He found it almost impossible to maintain a clear picture of what things had been like then. There had been no sulphone drugs, though chaulmoogra was being painfully injected and giving some hope and some real cures. There had been no prophetic word about emptying wards nor restored hands, no prospect of out-patient clinics which would take healing beyond the hospital. Yet what the bravest visionaries had not dared to predict was already reality. Though the war against leprosy showed no signs of being won – and twenty years later this would still be true – there had been some very notable victories indeed.

19: 'TLM' for Short
(1960–70)

By 1960 The Mission to Lepers was linked across much of Asia and Africa with a great variety of Protestant missions who were all committed to serving some of the most tragic people in the world. Over ninety different Christian societies and missions at work in more than thirty countries were helped by the Mission, and all this was in addition to the Mission's own homes and centres for which it was fully responsible. There were nearly thirty of these, all in Asia. The Mission's workers in its own stations, in addition to the large number of national workers, were truly international, from Asia, Australia, New Zealand, continental Europe and other countries in addition to those from Britain.

Now, alongside new drugs, new treatments and methods, and new successes, the Mission had other excitements to share with its supporters. Throughout this decade the Mission went on moving out into territories new to it, some of which subscribers might at first find hard to pin-point on the map. Siam had become Thailand. The Dutch East Indies were now Indonesia. What had we used to call Tanzania, Zaire or Zambia? How many people in Britain had ever heard of 'the Near North' where the Mission would be at work in the middle of the decade. Some of these new 'entries' will be briefly taken up in later chapters; all that follows here is an indication of the Mission's astonishing programme of expansion.

Hong Kong, at least, had a familiar sound, for it had been part of the British Empire for a century. Now it was the only British toe-hold left in China. When Wilfrid Russell made his 1962 tour of Asia he found, of course, very few of today's ubiquitous Rolls-Royces and Mercedes, and the sky-scraper business-city still lay in the future. Russell was much more aware of the thousands of refugees from China who crossed the border and found some sort of home in the shanty-towns they threw up wherever they could find space. But he also heard of the ten-year-old Hong Kong Auxiliary's recent Christmas fair which had raised £5000 to support a remarkable new project. This was Hay Ling Chau, the 'Isle of Happy Healing' – where an indomitable Mission to Lepers doctor had created a busy leprosarium, on an island that nobody wanted, for sufferers whom nobody wanted in Hong Kong itself. By the 1960s it had some 600 patients.

Relationships between The Mission to Lepers and national governments had changed greatly over the years and this was very clear when Russell visited Korea, well to the north of Hong Kong. At Taegu, where the Mission had worked some fifty years earlier, there was a Medical School where government doctors were trained and a Medical College Hospital in which their practical work was done. Dr Lee, the Dean, and Dr Sun, the Superintendent of the Hospital, explained to Russell their plans for the future – a big government hospital alongside the Medical School. It could include a leprosy section, suggested the Korean doctors, if The Mission to Lepers could provide the funds! A leprosy centre in the college grounds – with wards for in-patients, an out-patient department, an operating theatre and a physiotherapy unit . . . the Koreans began to fill out the details of their vision. By the following year it was well on its way to reality.

Back in India the General Secretary had an even more exciting date in his diary – not a discussion about new buildings, but the newest of all the Mission's hospitals. And that in a land which for centuries had been largely a 'closed country' – Nepal. The capital of this fascinating country is

Kathmandu, with narrow streets and busy bazaars, centuries-old temples and the palace of the sacred ruler himself, then King Mahendra. Not far from Kathmandu, in a valley brilliant green with rice-fields and guarded by the towering Himalayas, was a new building. It took its name from the pine-forest on the hill-slopes where it was built—Anandaban, 'the Forest of Joy'. This was the most recent of the hospitals of The Mission to Lepers, the only leprosy hospital in the state and here, on 23 November, 1963, the General Secretary joined medical staff and a crowd of expectant Nepalis for the official opening of the hospital.

In the same year another Government showed its appreciation of The Mission to Lepers. This was a long way from Nepal, amongst the deep green bush and red earth of southern Africa, in what was then Tanganyika, now Tanzania. Dr Neil Fraser, who had ferried the first boat-load of patients to the island of Hay Ling Chau, had visited Africa and offered useful guidance about the siting of a hospital at Hombolo, where the missionary-manager was an Australian, supported by the New Zealand auxiliary. The site, near a reservoir, gave a new complex its name—The Living Water Centre. It would be the base for a comprehensive leprosy service reaching out into the country over hundreds of square miles of bush and mountainous territory. Though not a Mission-based project it was an excellent example of the way Mission-support was now being given in Africa.

The following year attention switched back to the Himalayas to another country which through the years had also been firmly independent of 'foreign interest'. This was Bhutan. From the Prime Minister came an urgent invitation to The Mission to Lepers to help with the leprosy situation in that country. Eddie Askew, an able and distinguished layman who had already led Purulia to new achievements, was asked to visit Bhutan and 'report back'.

This he did with two Indian colleagues, but it sounded easier than it turned out to be. He described the visit in the Mission's magazine.

'Until two years ago there were only mule tracks from the border to the administrative capital, Paro, and the journey took six days trekking over steep, jungle-covered mountains inhabited by bears, elephants and leeches . . . Now there is a road, built with incredible skill by Indian army engineers, with Bhutanese and Nepali labourers . . . It claws its way up mountain-sides, clings to the face of sheer cliffs, teeters over 9,000-foot passes, nowhere more than sixteen feet wide and often much narrower. We had a journey to remember!' Beyond the passes they entered a narrow valley, widening out on each side of the icy river flowing down from the glaciers high in the mountains only thirty miles from Tibet. They found beauty, splendour, primitive living conditions – and leprosy everywhere. The invitation from the Bhutan Prime Minister was interpreted as a new call from God.

It was in this decade, too, that under Dr Paul Brand's inspiration, investigation went forward in Africa and ALERT, the All-Africa Leprosy Rehabilitation and Training Centre, was set up in Ethiopia, at Addis Ababa.

Mr Newberry Fox took over from Wilfrid Russell as General Secretary in 1965 and it was during this period that 'the Near North' began to appear more and more frequently in reports and magazine articles. Papua New Guinea – PNG for short – had become part of the British Empire in 1888 and had been handed over to Australia for administrative purposes in 1906. It was rugged, mountainous, broken by swift rivers, with important mineral deposits and natural resources, but until well after World War II it was almost totally unexplored and much of the Central Highlands were inaccessible. By that time inroads had been made into the bush, however, and aircraft could land in the Highlands. With the invading forces of commerce came

103

other people with deeper compassion. By the mid-1960s, when there were thirteen leprosy centres set up by as many different missionary societies, the expertise of The Mission to Lepers was called upon to offer training in remedial surgery and lead the way towards new life for patients who, more than in most places, were severely incapacitated.

In 1968, the Australian and New Zealand Auxiliaries took up a second challenge in another part of 'the Near North'. 'We propose to recruit a surgeon, a theatre sister, a physiotherapist and a business manager to set up a base settlement at Sitanala, about sixteen miles from Jakarta . . . and begin the same sort of work in Indonesia as we have done in Papua New Guinea.' By the end of the 1970s work had begun at Sitanala and a highly-skilled doctor had arrived from India to lead the surgical team.

In the midst of all these advances and changes, however, one thing about the Mission had remained the same.

The Mission to Lepers in India had, in 1893, become The Mission to Lepers in India and the East. It had been changed to The Mission to Lepers in 1913. And under that title it had continued for some fifty years. It had been generally agreed that 'leper' was a degrading word, which had been rejected first by the World Health Organization, then by the American Leprosy Mission and later outlawed by various national governments and agencies. A consultation of Mission workers held in the Isle of Wight in 1962 made it clear that for them, too, representing many countries in the world, the time for change had come. Medical opinion was strongly in favour of a new name. Despite some resistance from insensitive supporters a careful search had gone on for a suitable new title, and one was finally agreed.

Almost ninety years after its creation Wellesley Bailey's compassionate foundation became, quite simply, The Leprosy Mission.

It would be known, more familiarly, as TLM, for short.

20: The Fight Against Leprosy: 'Search and Destroy' (1960s onwards)

The Mission's report for 1969 reminded readers that it was exactly a hundred years since Wellesley Bailey first saw a group of leprosy sufferers in Ambala. 'Now', said the Report, contrasting past and present, 'places are available in our Indian hospitals for 10,000 patients. In the villages and out-patients clinics of the Indian hospitals more than 124,000 are receiving treatment.' That did not take account of the many other institutions outside India in which the Mission was in some way involved.

Even more impressive was the fact that in out-patient clinics posters were displayed with one simple, spectacular assertion.

'Leprosy can be cured!'

'And not only *can* be cured', said those who were pinning up the posters. 'It *is* being cured *now*.'

The really effective declaration came from those 'helpers' who went on to say something else. 'Look at me! *I* had leprosy and *I* am cured!'

But, impressive as all those things were, they did not present the whole truth.

A century after Bailey had begun his work there were still some 15,000,000 people in the world suffering from leprosy. And only one sufferer in every five was having any sort of treatment.

Despite all the posters and publicity, all the information broadcast by radio and all the news passed on by those who themselves were cured, it seemed that most people simply did not know that the disease was curable, that it was an ordinary disease like any other. Even in a country like India, wholly committed to the struggle, it appeared that more people were 'rescued' by accident than by design.

One such case was Padma, a girl of ten or eleven, who lived in a village in Orissa, an area where leprosy is rife. Everyone in her village, of course, believed it was a curse from the gods and Padma's family had seen one cursed already. Her mother Mugini had leprosy so badly that she could not walk on her damaged feet and she had been taken away on the back of a cycle to a nearby town. That had been years earlier and she had never come back, so the village felt itself to be free of the curse.

Then Mugini's husband, now with a new wife, saw the tell-tale signs in his daughter, Padma. The curse had *not* gone. He took Padma, too, to the town, Rairangpur, set her down in the street with a begging-bowl and cycled home.

Padma, mercifully, was picked up by kindly people and taken first to the Rairangpur clinic and from there was sent on to Mayurbhanj hospital. Though she could not understand why strangers should bother about her she was happy to have clean clothes, food and shelter, all of them better than she had known for a long time. She could do no more than wander about for a while, as she adjusted to the life of the hospital. Each evening she watched the women workers come back from the fields, able to walk, to plant and harvest the plants now that their feet and hands were so much restored. One of them passed Padma, listened to what she was saying, moved on and then came back to stare at her and clutch her in her arms.

Padma had been marvellously restored to her mother Mugini.

It was a splendid true story, almost made for publicity, with a happy ending – all the happier because both mother and daughter came to know Jesus, the healer. But it was not typical. Most children would not find their lost parents. Many would not even find their way to a clinic. And there were countless villages where thousand of Muginis and Padmas were hiding their tell-tale signs of leprosy.

It was to meet this world-wide situation of hidden or unrecognised leprosy that the next great campaign was organised. Espionage stories, so popular in our time, send out their secret agents with basically simple instructions. 'Search and Destroy!' The key-words of the new campaign were not dissimilar, and held the same implication. 'Survey . . . Education . . . Treatment.' SET for short.

This was not, of course, solely a Leprosy Mission concept. It arose from consultations, now a continuing part of the war on leprosy world-wide, between social agencies, missionary societies, government departments and international organisations such as the World Health Organization. The basic idea was simple – but very demanding in terms of staffing, finance and skills. Instead of waiting for the people to come to the village clinic *the health agencies would go to the people* – and not merely to those who were known to have, or might have, the disease but to *everybody*. Those who were found to have leprosy, however early the stage might be or however long they might have had it, would receive treatment. And everyone would be taught about it. The plan was crystallised in a striking headline in *New Day*, The Leprosy Mission's new magazine.

'The Leprosy Mission Takes On Three Million!' said the title. The article opened: 'A major "growth area" of the Mission today is the setting up of Survey-Education-Treatment schemes in the new areas. The Government of India is asking the Mission to play a greater part in the nation's fight against leprosy . . . and to take on *four* areas with a total population of three million!'

From the government's standpoint this was a massive attack on a disease that had so far proved unconquerable. In the Mission's view it was more than this. 'The aim is to make this work an effective piece of Christian witness as well as employing one of the latest methods of leprosy

107

control'. This did not mean 'overt attempts at conversion' but meant that everything Christian workers did, and their attitudes to those they dealt with would be a commendation of the Lord whom they served. The fact that they did what they did in the way they did ought, in itself, to demonstrate Christ's compassion as well as medical skill. It was a token of official confidence in the Mission's stance that considerable numbers of Indian government workers were sent to the Mission's hospitals and centres for training.

How did SET work?

Even on the massive scale envisaged by the Indian Government it was simply an extension of what The Leprosy Mission had been doing for some time, and examples provide a clear picture of what had been happening.

'We got one room at Daryabad – an old, dilapidated room but on the main road – and patients have started to come. During the rains it leaks so much that we have to sit under our umbrellas, and the road is so bad that in the rains it takes us an hour to cover six miles.'

That was a fair description of many ordinary out-patient clinics. At the Jhalda Control Unit the three elements of SET, based on the wayside clinic, are clearer. Four students went out with the physiotherapist to conduct 'roadside clinics'. That was precisely what they were – places where the Unit's jeep pulled up by the roadside and got to work. For trainee physiotherapy technicians 'working at the roadside certainly developed powers of imagination and initiative. Posters were hung on the side of the jeep. Booklets on handcare and footcare were displayed by propping them up against ant-hills. And patients did hand-massage and exercise, squatting on a long strip of plastic on a soft patch of grass, anchored against the wind by a few stones.' And then on to similar clinics, and more the next day, and the days after that.

Though Education and Treatment are obvious in such an

example, the great importance of the para-medical workers must not be forgotten. One of these PMWs, as they were known, was later featured in a TLM film made in 1976. Even as late as that, in *The Net*, Joseph did not look very much like a key figure! He was a slim Indian Christian villager with a bicycle on which he might travel fifty or sixty miles along rough roads and tracks. One of hundreds of paramedical workers on the Mission's books he represented a new corps of shock-troops in the anti-leprosy campaign. PMWs, both men and women, whether employed by missions or governments, were given a careful training which enabled them to detect leprosy in its early stages as well as recognising its more obvious forms. PMWs were trained to take 'smears' from such 'suspects' and these were passed to the laboratory for examination. The PMW also carried medication, including anti-leprosy pills; gave instructions about dosage; and kept records of all patients. Employed to keep in touch with the population in a specific area PMWs were equipped to provide regular oversight of those who could be treated at home, to help base hospitals or control centres to build up 'surveys' of a wide area, and to arrange for those who needed special treatment to be taken to hospital.

PMWs were basically 'skilled people from amongst the people themselves'. Without them the whole SET programme would have collapsed. The programme, however, also demanded techniques and knowledge which the PMW could not be expected to possess.

While the rural PMW might well be able to talk to the small village school which gathered under the village trees, larger and more formal schools expected better-equipped visitors. One South Indian missionary reports that 'PMWs have completed approximately two-thirds of the Survey in the project area.' He then goes on: 'Every school in the project area has been visited at least once, several more than once, and talks given to pupils and staff.' Flannelgraphs and posters were popular in village-visits and in schools, but in addressing school staffs and upper forms in high schools the presentation and expectation had to be more professional, and the questions would demand very competent answers.

'Education' also implied equipping 'leaders'. In one town a 'laymen's teaching class' was held for a day with ten village leaders and six schoolteachers. In another there was a whole week's course on 'how to get the message across' – and in that week a dozen simple plays were written, rehearsed and acted, all good enough to be taken on tour in the villages, often to be performed by women, and all would communicate as effectively as formal talks. Village leaders, teachers and church workers would go back from such courses to dispel the traditional fear of leprosy and encourage people to come forward for treatment.

There was a still more highly-organised method of 'survey' where whole teams of workers were mobilised and sent to selected areas, usually where PMWs had already been at work. Jeeps and land-rovers; vehicles spilling out folding-tables, boxes of medicines; tents; nurse; record-keeper; footwear specialist; smear technician; physiotherapist . . . as all these set up camp under their mango-trees it must have seemed to the villagers that the hospital itself had materialised in their midst. There would be material for village after-work talk for months to come. With the authority of the headman the whole village would be paraded; howling babies and aged men and women were not exempt. All the school-children would be examined. The day's work which, if it were organised by a Mission, would have begun with a Bible-reading and prayer would end in the same way. But, by that time, among the hundreds of villagers and school-children examined, perhaps a score or more of people who had leprosy – often in its very elementary form – would have been discovered. For each of them the promise was that they would not be excluded or segregated.

One of the great pioneers, Dr Ernest Muir, had said long

before: 'If we are going to conquer leprosy we must go to the place where leprosy begins . . . to the village'. SET was putting into action that eager and driving vision. In villages across the plains of India, in the paddy-fields of Thailand and Indonesia, among the red hills and along the red roads of Africa, in the mountains on the coastal villages of Papua New Guinea, under the towering Himalayas in Nepal and Bhutan, mobile teams of lonely paramedical workers, many of them linked with The Leprosy Mission, carried hope to the people.

21: A Year of Grace (1974)

1974 was the centenary year of the Mission.

It was a year that had seen frustrations and disappointments as well as having a great many reasons for thanksgiving. China was still a closed country in which leprosy-work, if it existed at all, was in no way linked with the missions which had pioneered it. Burmese frontiers allowed only a thin trickle of news through from Kin Thein and his wife Ruth, who had been the first physiotherapist working with Dr Paul Brand in south India. Moulmein, they said, was the only one of the old Mission stations still active, though the high cost of food had reduced the number of patients from 225 to 146. Government leprosy controls were at work but that meant no more visits by the Christian workers to villages and no direct access by the hospital to rural areas. In this Buddhist country with its Socialist leadership, however, it was something to thank God for that church-services in the hospital were well-attended and the choir was enthusiastic!

Other things in the overseas reports had become predictable. SET – making surveys, educating workers and more particularly the people themselves, treating early cases through the widening use of paramedical workers – all this appeared in one report after another. Mysore wrote about 'a SET programme with four PMWs covering sixty-four villages.' Vadala, in Maharashtra, quoted 'an intensive survey that dealt with 188,725 people'. In Kothara it was only 110,000 people! Yet a few years earlier even two or three thousand people examined for leprosy in one sweeping survey would have seemed almost incredible.

Implicit in many of the Indian reports was the steady breaking-down of fear and prejudice. 'We are getting many more high-class patients' . . . 'The out-patients' department draws teachers, students, farmers, policemen, army personnel, businessmen.' . . . 'We had an "Open Day" and it was surprising how many people ventured to come'. It had not been so long ago that such people would have hesitated to admit they had leprosy and would have hesitated even more to touch someone they knew to have the disease.

Now 'touching people' was not so frightening. Dichpalli was one centre where 'touching' was very deliberate policy! There, patients were keen on sport and especially on cricket and football. But why should leprosy patients only play against fellow-patients? Uneasily and then with enthusiasm local village teams first played cricket and then football with the hospital. And what closer contact could one expect than on the football field?

There was indeed a great deal to thank God for in this centenary year. Not least was this true of names which, not long previously, were not even on The Leprosy Mission's books. There were success stories from Nepal—leprosy workers becoming involved in the general medical service in Bhutan—leprosy patients accepted in general hospitals in Sumatra—two Finnish nurses on TLM staff, working in a thirty-five-bed leprosy ward in a general hospital in Java—leprosy work being integrated into the general health service in Papua New Guinea. There were new names in Africa, too—nearly forty stations in fourteen countries, all given help by The Leprosy Mission, and all sending reports which matched those from India and the rest of Asia.

The annual published report usually included stories which brought unfamiliar situations to life . . . stories about workers, for instance, like the Australian nurse and her colleague setting off for a seven day tour in northern Thailand. Nothing 'touristic' about this tour, though—it was to run the regular village clinics which depended on such visits month by month. They set off at 6.00 in the morning, in the cool time of the day, and after four and a half hours driving were just two miles away from the leprosy village on the other side of the river. The only problem was that half the bridge had been washed away – and the half that remained was attached to the further bank of the river. Leaving the landrover on the muddy bank the two nurses managed to find a partly-submerged plank, slithered across it to the other side, and walked the two kilometres to the village. Only one patient turned up for examination.

Back to the river, across the slimy plank, into the Landrover with its precious cargo of medicines and then, partly along the way they had already come, another three and a half hours rough driving before they reached another road. The detour would add another five hours to their first day's journey – and there were six more days to follow. Like many of their colleagues in Africa and Asia and the Pacific these nurses had learned to take the rough with the smooth, and accept that there is not likely to be many straightforward events on a week's trek through the village clinics. There was still more in store on this first day of the tour, for they had only gone three kilometres when they passed over another rough bridge of logs. Or, more accurately, half-passed over it, for the front wheel slipped off the round, slimy tree-trunks and down between them with the back wheel ready to follow. It took hours of eager work by helpful Thais, all shouting at the tops of their voices, before the Landrover was safely on the other side of the river. Not until 8.00 in the evening did they reach their first day's destination.

The Report editor could have found plenty of other stories like that, for 'things happened' to leprosy workers all over the world all through the year! But readers would want to have stories of leprosy *patients*, too, and there were many that cried out for inclusion.

One was from Medan, in Sumatra, Indonesia, about a filthy beggar who crawled into the clinic on, what was left of its hands and knees. Man or woman, boy or girl? It was impossible to tell until the nurses had picked him up, washed

114

him clean and put him in a bed. For the previous month this young man had been living in a gutter, existing on scraps that he found among the garbage. For seventeen years he had been begging in the Medan streets, where his father had brought him from his village when he was ten years old and dumped him on the pavement.

Before that, and before his father had discovered that he had leprosy, the boy had been to school and it became clear that nearly twenty years in the gutters had not quite robbed him of the ability to read and write. The Leprosy Mission sister found him reading a copy of the Indonesian translation of *The Upper Room*. It was the beginning of a new road to hope and healing.

From Africa came a different kind of story about SET. In Zambia a paramedical worker had made arrangements for the hospital's survey team to visit a village where he had come across ten suspected leprosy cases and a number of other people needing medical treatment. When the team arrived the sight was extraordinary. About a hundred villagers were busily at work. They had already started building a mud dispensary to be ready for the hospital team. Now some were completing the walls and others putting in timber for the roof. Women were levelling the ground round the building. They were eager to welcome the team and even more eager to sit down first and listen to the stories of Jesus, though only a few of them were already Christians. Not surprisingly, perhaps, the dispensary was the prelude to more building – the erection of a tiny church. No story would better illustrate the contribution of paramedical workers throughout Africa and Asia, the way their primary task of offering ways to health was matched by the happy commendation of Jesus as Saviour. If it was a very simple gospel it was received by simple people with gladness.

The same emphasis was found in many of the letters on the editor's desk, and matched by the way staff members in hospitals shared in leading prayers in wards and services in chapel; the story of the hospital chaplain who gave gospel teaching in eight wayside SET clinics; and the account of a Punjabi hospital where the patients, illiterate and one of them blind, enthusiastically formed a drama group to present the Christian message.

At Taegu, in Korea, they had decided to celebrate the 'centenary year' by increasing the number of out-station educational visits to one hundred, too. These included schools and village visits, and the villages varied greatly in their reception of the 'education team'. Sometimes the weather was bone-chilling cold, at others dusty and hot. The welcomes were just as varied – from warm to dull to cold! In 5,000 miles of travel they presented educational programmes in village squares, village halls – and village graveyards! But, so the report from Korea stated: '30,000 people learned more about leprosy – and about Jesus.'

A note of hope ran through the whole year's work . . . not only of hope, indeed, but of achievement.

A hundred years earlier Charlotte Pim in Dublin had transformed a promise of 'perhaps £30 a year' into an actual sum of £600 to help Wellesley Bailey in his work in north India. *In the centenary year The Leprosy Mission's income was £1,214,000 – the first time it had broken through the million pound barrier, and it was thirty-five per cent higher than the previous year!*

Fifty years earlier, at the Jubilee Thanksgiving Service, Wellesley Bailey had spoken out of his own experience. 'The Mission is "a building not made with hands". God has been the builder, and because of that fact . . . it has gone on prospering and *will* prosper!' And God's grace had not only been sufficient for those early years; it had been sufficient for the Mission through *all* the years. *Every* year had been a year of grace.

It was under that title that the Centenary Report of The Leprosy Mission went out to subscribers and supporters.

The Centenary Year had indeed been *'A Year of Grace'*.

22: The Fight Against Leprosy: Battle Stations: Report from Bergen (1973)

1973 was the centenary of Armauer Hansen's discovery of the leprosy bacillus, and in that hundred years the leprosy scene had changed beyond recognition. The first fifty years of frustrated research had given place first to the chaulmoogra period and then to the sulphone era, with dapsone as the cheapest and best form of the new drug. No one now seemed hesitant to use the word 'cure'. Leprosy workers used it in their reports and patients went back from hospital and clinic proclaiming it exultantly.

It was all true. People *were* cured. They went into the world with new hands and feet, new faces, even new – if artificial – arms and legs, too.

But, in fact, not everything was quite so triumphantly successful as it sounded.

In 1973 the Tenth Congress of the International Leprosy Association was held, appropriately, in Bergen. There were over a thousand members of the Congress from more than eighty countries, representing all branches of medical science, all the main divisions of the Christian church, governments from five continents and many international organisations. Over 370 papers had been submitted for presentation to the Congress, and they ranged from high-powered techniques in the laboratory to rehabilitation of leprosy patients. The mood was one of restrained optimism for in the past two or three decades there had been greater advances in knowledge and practice, treatment and social renewal, than at any period in the century.

There were, however, speakers who swept away any sense of euphoria.

'We have on our hands a *new* problem; a more intractable problem than we have had before. It is not only that there are more people in the world suffering from leprosy than we had realised. But people whom we had thought to be cured are *not* always cured!'

None of the discussion undervalued the astonishing contribution of DDS; it had done more than anything else to cure leprosy sufferers. But those who had been treated, and were now free of symptoms, would need to continue the dapsone treatment to maintain that freedom, some for months, some for years and some for life.

One story illustrated the point very clearly. A young African, educated and in good employment, discovered that he had signs of leprosy. If this became generally known he would be finished in his profession and in his marriage prospects, but fortunately he heard of a 'skin clinic' where he might get help. The inoffensive name was deliberate. Since a public visit might expose his condition he made private arrangements to consult one of the staff. His fears proved right; he *did* have leprosy – *but*, and this he could hardly believe, it could be cured! It meant regular visits for check-ups, daily doses of dapsone, careful and disciplined living. In a few months the signs had gone. It was only just in time for he was soon due to be married and he could not have faced the possibility of his wife's finding the signs of the disease.

'You must keep on coming back for check-ups,' they said at the clinic.

But he couldn't do that. His wife might find out.

'You must certainly keep on taking the tablets. If you give them up the leprosy may come back. And you must come back here for the tablets regularly.'

The young man shook his head. He had *had* leprosy, but

it was gone. He could not risk being seen at the clinic again.

When he had gone the workers shook their heads in despair. They had done half a job, but not a whole job; the other half had to be done by the patients themselves. They had told this man the truth. He was cured but that did not mean the germ was conquered. Unless, in his case, he kept on taking the tablets month after month, year after year, the disease would recur.

And – this was the hardest part of the truth that was only now becoming apparent – if it *did* recur it might not be curable by going back on the drug. Experience was showing that leprosy germs were developing their own resistance to the powerful drugs now in use. From all over the world there were reports of patients relapsing even after prolonged treatment. What was still more disturbing, if lepromatous patients who had relapsed passed on the disease those who were infected were likely to be themselves resistant to the dapsone and incapable of effective treatment.

The leprosy workers and scientists at the Bergen Congress were called to battle-stations once again.

Dr Stanley Browne, the great Central Africa missionary who had become The Leprosy Mission's Medical Consultant, put it concisely. 'Things are getting worse. We must look for new and more effective drugs. We have two or three good ones, but one of them costs about £200 per person per year. And that's quite out of the question for a Christian Mission trying to treat some 450,000 people in the world today.'

It was to be another ten years before The Leprosy Mission took its next momentous step in the use of new and more hopeful drugs.

But, meanwhile, the work went on.

23: The Isle of Happy Healing – Hong Kong (1951–75)

The next few chapters pick up and expand the references in chapter twenty to the new areas in which The Leprosy Mission began work during the 1950s and '60s. Much of the interest, apart from the work itself, lies in the differing ways in which the Mission was offered openings which it was happy to accept after careful investigation – openings which came from governments as well as from churches and missions, which made growing financial demands and challenged both the faith of the Mission's officers and the commitment of an expanding number of supporters and workers in many countries.

The Leprosy Mission had, for the greater part of its existence, been an international organisation and had become more so through the years. Now it was very demonstrably so. The pattern of the 1950s and '60s has been maintained so that by the 1980s some forty TLM missionaries, all of them medical, were at work in the countries first 'entered' in that period. They came from America and Canada; from Australia, New Zealand and Japan; from Europe – Belgium, Denmark, Finland, France, Germany, Holland and Switzerland; from Ireland and Great Britain. Year by year the list of people and countries changes a little but the skills remain high and the motive the same, one of Christian compassion.

This chapter takes up the beginning of the Mission's work in Hong Kong. And, for once, it is a story that has an end, too.

In Hong Kong both government and Mission became aware of a growing problem. Dr Neil Fraser, one of the Mission's experienced leprosy workers, had been at work in China but like other westerners was compelled to leave when Chairman Mao's government was established. Over the same period many Chinese moved across the border into over-crowded Hong Kong, settling into squatter quarters under the shadow of the Peak or where they could find space in Kowloon.

It became apparent to the Hong Kong medical authorities that among the massive influx of workless, homeless and often sick people there were many suffering from leprosy which, in China, was regarded as an affliction from the gods as a result of an evil or immoral life. Those who suffered from it were often driven away. To Dr Fraser the situation suggested both a problem and an opportunity which ought not to be neglected.

The Hong Kong government had, in the past, maintained a small leprosy hospital but it was becoming apparent that a much larger leprosarium would now be needed. Dr Fraser reported to London when he visited the Mission's headquarters and he returned to Hong Kong with full support for 'doing what was necessary'. The colony's government interpreted 'what was necessary' as segregation – and as isolated as possible on one of the colony's many islands. To this policy, and especially to an island leprosarium, Fraser objected very strongly – but without effect.

There are few more lovely seascapes in Asia than Hong Kong. Hilly and flat, bare or tree-covered, large and small, dotted with fisher-families' villages, the islands are everywhere. Fraser's problem was that if he found an island that seemed suitable the local inhabitants objected to the idea of leprosy sufferers coming among them. He sought through the blue sea, under the azure sky and became increasingly frustrated until he came on the uninhabited Nun Island. But it was uninhabited because there was no fresh water.

The authorities, with the possibility of segregation becoming a reality, proved more co-operative. When Fraser found a spring of fresh water the army sent a party of Royal Engineers who made a fuller survey and provided a constant and splendid water-supply. The Hong Kong government made grants for the first hospital-buildings, and both the Mission and the government provided grants for the development of the island. The churches in Hong Kong recognised the situation as a challenge to themselves, too, and the Hong Kong Auxiliary of the Mission was established. It was to provide a continual flow of funds for the hospital and, as time went on, would be the base from which pastoral and social care would be offered to those who were discharged from treatment on the island. Its committee was widely representative of the Hong Kong community.

The venture became an outstanding success, and became one of the Mission's notable achievements.

In August 1951 Dr Neil Fraser sailed from the wharves of Hong Kong in a boat with four courageous men, the first pioneers and patients of the new enterprise. They weaved between large and small islands until, nine miles from the city of Hong Kong itself, they reached Nun Island and, with their coming, its transformation began. The sign of it was the new name given to the island – Hay Ling Chau, 'the Isle of Happy Healing'. Soon after the arrival of Fraser's first patients the hospital buildings began to rise. In its first year, with accommodation for 300 patients, the reputation of Hay Ling Chau began to spread not only through Hong Kong but into mainland China. In 1954 the Hospital was officially opened by the Governor of Hong Kong and was named the 'Maxwell Memorial Hospital' after a veteran leprosy doctor from China who was now a Vice-President of the Mission. To the Chinese people, of course, the name mattered little. It was simply the happy island where people with leprosy were astonishingly given back their health and often the use of their limbs. As sufferers began to comprehend that leprosy was not an affliction from unseen powers but was an ordinary disease which, at Hay Ling Chau, was being cured there came a steady stream of eager and sometimes desperate patients.

They were directed there by the government medical clinics in Hong Kong and Kowloon and came from every level of society and at every stage of the disease. The only thing many of then had in common was despair.

Yellow Jade was one of them, and not untypical. Her story was published in a booklet about Hay Ling Chau and its earlier patients. Her uncle, who lived in the family home when she was a little girl, was turned out of the house when it was discovered that he had contracted leprosy. Yellow Jade would never forget the day she joined with other children in jeering at him, or the following morning when it was found he had hanged himself. She herself came to the same kind of despair. Married at eighteen and a mother soon afterwards she had known of the patches on her arm for years and kept them hidden. Then, soon after her baby died, her husband died also, and the patches began to appear on her face and she could no longer hide them. Like her uncle, she was driven away.

By accident, in a tea-house she overheard some young men talking of an island in Hong Kong where leprosy sufferers could be cured, and Yellow Jade became determined to try and reach the great city, a hundred miles away beyond the Chinese frontier. She had little money and received little charity, except from the old and the poor, but at the end of a month's walking she crossed the border and was swallowed up in the raucous complex of Hong Kong. At the end of the day, with nowhere to go, she crawled up some house-steps and dropped into an exhausted sleep in a corner of a verandah. There, next morning, she was wakened by an angry servant who was driving her away when the house-owner came out. An Indian, he listened compassionately to her story, gave her food and ensured that she was given the chance of going to the island hospital.

Month by month there came people like Yellow Jade,

people with histories of rejection, fear and desolation. There were young boys and girls, old men and women; shopkeepers, hairdressers and clerks; seamen and mothers with children holding on to hand or skirt. For them all there was a welcome, treatment suited to their special needs, and in most cases work was given to them which in some measure restored their self-respect. Additional government grants increased the capacity of the hospital to 540 beds.

A visitor described the journey from Hong Kong island to Hay Ling Chau in The Leprosy Mission's own motor-vessel, the *Ling Hong*, and how she found it a place of beauty and busy activity. First, from the boat, was the sight of green vegetable fields, pine woods and sandy beaches. Then, beyond the stone jetty, the brilliant flame-of-the-forest trees with their scarlet flowers and, up the roadway, the scattered buildings of the leprosarium. 'Attractive stone cottages and workshops for the patients, a valley with fields and terraces, agricultural areas and careful irrigation ... busy and active people everywhere – farmers, gardeners, pig- and duck-keepers, carpenters, plumbers, bean-curd-makers, cobblers, electricians. There were wood-carvers, too, and model-makers ... barbers and boatmen.' It was a description not of an old-fashioned static hospital or a shut-off segregated community, but of a very different kind of leprosarium – a village which, in its activities and life-style, could be matched anywhere in China.

At the heart of the village was an interdenominational church with a Chinese Lutheran pastor, and while only a minority of the patients were Christians there were always some who found new life and fulfilment in Christ while they were there. The international foreign staff, as well as the Chinese, made their own witness with life and word. Some men, having become Christians, went on after leaving the island to train as evangelists and preachers at the Lutheran Bible School.

Year after year the healing work of Hay Ling Chau continued and its development matched the changing pattern of leprosy work in the rest of the world. The new drugs brought speedier relief. Seemingly hopeless people with drapped feet, clawed hands or collapsed noses entered a new world of mobility and activity after surgery and physiotherapy. The length of time needed for hospital treatment grew constantly shorter.

Nevertheless, for many of the patients there were problems when they left the island. In Hong Kong itself, where the old folk-image of leprosy persisted among many people, discharged and cured patients were treated with suspicion, or with contempt because they had once had the disease. It was not easy to be rehabilitated. Nevertheless, enough made good to give courage to others who left – and some did very well indeed. There was the barber who went back to his old profession, opened a small shop, did well enough to open a larger one, and sent to Hay Ling Chau to take on another ex-patient as his assistant. A sea-going engineer became a Christian while he was under treatment. He looked, they said, like a water-pirate, but he wanted to stay on when he was ready for discharge to repay by hard work some of the kindness shown to him. He was no landsman and in the end went back to the engine-rooms of the big ships on the Pacific trade-routes.

One of the first four men who came to the island with Dr Fraser was chosen with prayer and great care to lead the first 'resettlement party' to leave the island, a man of integrity and faith who was a leader in the little Hay Ling Chau Christian community. With three other men he was to try and settle in a village called Taai Pak where they would help to create a new community. The patients said goodbye and waited for news. They had not long to wait! The next Sunday all four men were back again! But they did not come seeking re-admission; they stood up in the service to tell of the way they had been accepted, given work and a certain measure of friendship. For those with courage there was often a way back into the world beyond the island.

From the beginning there had been a rather inadequate

church building on Hay Ling Chau – 'The Lord is Willing' church – but plans for a more worthy one became reality in 1966 when the lovely new church was opened. The paradoxical situation was that not long after the new church was opened there was already talk of the possible end of Hay Ling Chau leprosarium. For years the number of patients remained steady at 540. Then, gradually, it began to fall and by 1968 it had dropped to 281. This was not due, of course, to any failure in the work of The Leprosy Mission in the hospital but, on the contrary, to its new success. The changes in treatment, the new criteria for discharge, the effect of the reconstructive surgery programme, and the continued development of out-patient clinics in Hong Kong itself were responsible for the island's work being run down. Almost as significant was the change in atmosphere which Hay Ling Chau had helped to generate – a new attitude of 'acceptance' developed as it was demonstrated that the disease was a natural one and not nearly so infectious as, for instance, the common cold or influenza. In some cases those who had leprosy could work and live in normal society, or attend school or college, without providing a threat to their neighbours, and could certainly do so after treatment.

The Hong Kong authorities at last accepted what other countries had already practised – that 'segregation' was not an essential element in contemporary treatment of the disease. Once that had been recognised the policy of leprosy sufferers being incarcerated on an island 'a safe distance from the city' was abandoned.

In 1970 the Hong Kong government agreed plans for a splendid new medical complex at Lai Chai Kok which was to be known as the Princess Margaret Hospital and, while it would be a general hospital for the citizens of the Colony, it would also include an infectious diseases ward for leprosy and other patients and those undergoing reconstructive surgery. Most leprosy sufferers would not need to be admitted to a hospital at all and would find the help they needed, with the necessary drugs and advice, in out-patient clinics.

By January 1975 Hay Ling Chau's ministry was over. At special ceremonies long-service awards were presented to Chinese staff-members who now had to make new lives for themselves. The Isle of Happy Healing had exercised a ministry of some twenty-five years which, in the history of The Leprosy Mission, was unique. The outstanding co-operation of the Mission, the government, the community and the churches had brought hope and healing to thousands of people in the Colony and from mainland China, and for many of them Jesus Christ the great healer had himself become a transforming reality.

Though in no way associated with The Leprosy Mission, Hay Ling Chau is now a government centre for the treatment of drug addicts.

24: Into the Himalayas
– Nepal and Bhutan
(1957 onwards)

It may have implied very useful public recognition that The Leprosy Mission could work in close co-operation with government as it did in Hong Kong, even though officialdom lagged behind the Mission in its ideas, but there were even more remarkable overtures in this period – an appeal from a Prime Minister and an invitation from a King! True, their kingdoms were remote, but they were certainly romantic! These invitations to begin work in the Himalayan states of Nepal and Bhutan represented a new kind of breakthrough in the Mission's outreach for they were both 'closed' countries to the outside world through the centuries, both by policy and by the sheer physical difficulties of getting into them. Conversion from one faith to another was firmly discouraged, but Christian missionaries had already, on limited terms, been accepted.

It was in Nepal, where the summit of Everest had been scaled only four years previously by Hilary and Tensing Sherpa, that the Mission was, in 1957, offered some thirty acres of land not far from the capital, Kathmandu. Barriers were already being taken down. While Christian missionaries as evangelistic agents were still excluded the king was deeply concerned that his hill-kingdom should not be deprived of the benefits of the modern world. Education, medical and social services, and some relief of the leprosy problem, would all be welcome and as agents of these progressive reforms

Christian missionaries – provided they did not set out to proselytise – were welcomed too.

Six years after land had been granted to the Mission the new hospital for leprosy patients was built. Named Anandaban, 'the Forest of Joy', its erection had involved considerable problems, including the transport of material over almost impassable roads and lifting water several hundred feet from the stream at the base of the hillside. On Saturday, 23 November, 1963, King Mahendra was to declare the hospital open. That day, however, the world was shocked by the news of the assassination of President Kennedy; the court went into mourning and the opening was carried out in the king's absence. He did, however, make an official visit with the queen some months later at a striking public occasion.

A few years later the royal family became still further involved with leprosy work. Nepal health officials had shared in a consultation about the disease with other countries and the World Health Organization, and in 1969, with one of the royal princesses as its active chairman, the Nepal Leprosy Relief Association was founded. Public opinion about the disease began to change and amendments to the laws made leprosy work both easier to conduct and more accessible to even the more remote sufferers.

Three years later in The Leprosy Mission's official report there were references which reflected some of these changes in attitude and service. The report's unfamiliar names in the high mountain kingdom are not important; what is significant is the sense of activity, acceptance and hope which runs through it. 'An increase in new cases . . . over 100 operations performed . . . 356 new patients at the Shanta Bhawan clinic and 556 new ones at Jumla and the hospital clinics . . . the Anandaban hospital recognised as a referral centre and patients received from remote areas . . .' To those who thought of Nepal only as a mountaineers' paradise or a Shangri-la for 'hippies' this was a very different picture indeed.

But what did 'remote areas' really mean? A leprosy programme initiated in the largest of Nepal's fourteen 'zones' was remote indeed, but linked to the Anandaban hospital in the capital. Inaugurated by the Director of Health himself it involved two-hour plane flights over the Himalayan ranges. The beginning, of course, was a thorough-going survey in this high-incidence leprosy area. Sufferers in Karanali had already been making their way to Anandaban for treatment – for some of them that meant a thirty-day journey on foot into India, then by train back to Nepal and by bus to Kathmandu! For most hill-people such a journey was unthinkable and the new programme, beginning with two paramedical workers spending four months in the far-off zone, marked a new beginning of hope.

In different parts of the country, in co-operation with government and with other agencies such as the United Mission to Nepal, through clinics, surveys and research, and by providing training in crafts and skills such as in the farm created at Anandaban, The Leprosy Mission extended its work of hope and healing year by year.

'Druk', they who live there call it – 'Dragonland' – but on maps and atlases marked as 'Bhutan', it was the second Himalayan kingdom into which The Leprosy Mission was invited. The invitation in 1964 from the Prime Minister of Bhutan – a country smaller than Nepal, further to the east, but still bordering both India and Tibet – was urgent. The first response could be no more than a journey of investigation. It was undertaken by a team of three people working in India – two Indian doctors, P J Chandy and V P Das, and A D Askew, then at Purulia but soon to become the International Director of TLM. The narrow roads, high precipitous passes, slimy mud, deep and almost perpendicular gorges were in themselves sufficient to explain how 'the dragon state' had maintained its secrecy and isolation.

Now Bhutan was 'open' – if travellers were prepared to venture the new but still hazardous roads. Open, certainly to The Leprosy Mission, and a year after the Prime Minister's appeal, a German doctor and his wife were appointed in

1966 to take over a small hospital very recently opened at Gida Kom. He set out to discover as much as he could about the local people and to gain their confidence. The doctor spoke of '. . . a lot of touring, marching and climbing, by jeep, on foot, on horseback, with our only staff member who knows Bhutanese as companion.' The people themselves turned out to be friendly and very ready to 'show their hands and feet and backs with much laughing and joking', no doubt partly from embarrassment. Here and there sufferers had been overtly shunned, like the girl who had to 'live in a pigsty outside the village with herself in one compartment and the two pigs in the sty next door' though despite their enforced segregation by the community such situations were unusual. The doctor's tact and wisdom quickly broke down the barriers between expatriate staff and Bhutanese villagers and the hospital began to grow in size and numbers, with the full support and encouragement of government officials.

By 1967 there was a new hospital block ready for opening – and this, too, was a royal occasion with the Queen of Bhutan herself to untie the two silk scarves across the entrance to the building. It was, in fact, not a very large building! There were two rooms with eight beds in each for leprosy patients and two small rooms with two beds in each for general patients. Nevertheless the additional beds increased the capacity of the hospital to sixty patients and the new premises demonstrated very clearly the policy of the Mission, which in Bhutan, by agreement, was different from its work in many other places. The first doctors had quickly discovered that there was as much need for *general* medical care in this far-off region as there was for leprosy treatment. So, at Gida Kom in the following year there was still more building – a laundry, a central kitchen, and an X-ray room among other things. The year after that came an operating theatre and a recreation and occupational therapy room. There were fruit trees planted on the hillsides and farmland was cultivated around the hospital. Patients were admitted for general treatment as well as for leprosy, and many had to stay much longer than they would usually have done in small hospitals because travel and communication were so much more difficult than in states outside the Himalayas.

The Mission had seldom become so quickly and fully involved in a new situation as it did in Bhutan. But there was more to come.

In 1971 the Royal Government asked for a full-scale appreciation of the country's leprosy situation and the National Assembly passed a recommendation without amendment. 'If leprosy is to be brought under control we must establish a hospital in the East of the State.' The town of Mongar appeared the best choice. Would The Leprosy Mission be prepared to establish a hospital there? After careful consideration the Mission agreed to do so. It seemed that it might be possible to have a hospital functioning for general and leprosy patients by 1978 – seven years after the leprosy survey was suggested.

But occasionally things move quickly in the Himalayas! By 1975, three years ahead of schedule, the hospital at Mongar was open. The complex, with the main hospital and all the ancillary services, with the personal interest of the new king and the enthusiasm of the Legislative Assembly to support it, was quickly at work fighting many kinds of illness and disease. Leprosy patients came for treatment by drugs or for operations to restore their hands, their collapsed noses or their feet – but children were also brought with the killer-disease, measles, and the other killer, whooping cough. The leprosy sufferers, in particular, came long distances – from down in the valleys or up in the mountains. New patients were discovered as the result of surveys and old patients who had been treated in the west of the country at Gida Kom now made a day's march to show that they were fully recovered.

Mongar was the largest single investment The Leprosy Mission had ever made in Southern Asia – and one which might not have been expected in a Buddhist state which through the centuries had been closed to the rest of the world.

25: The Near North –
Papua New Guinea and
Indonesia (1974)

'The Near North'?

While Britain and Europe talk about the 'Far East' Americans think of Hong Kong or Korea as 'the West'. But to Australians and New Zealanders these are more like the 'Far North'. It depends where you live, for your centre of the world is *there*, as a rule. 'The Near North' is the Australian descriptive phrase for their huge neighbouring island, Papua New Guinea. The largest non-continental island in the world, only a hundred miles or so to the north of Austrlia, it was under Australian government by mandate from the League of Nations following World War I, when the territory ceased to be a German colony.

Papua New Guinea remained largely unknown even in the present century and its Central Highlands were almost completely unexplored. Only in the last quarter-century has 'white civilisation' for good or ill, broken into what was virtually a 'stone age society' so that now ancient and once-secret ceremonies are enacted for plane-loads of brash and insensitive tourists. Yet, by contrast, in the coastal areas there are big towns with all the 'modernity' of urban life while outside the towns mining, in particular, has eaten its way into the earth and the lives of these friendly and gracious Melanesian peoples.

The Australian authorities had a real concern for the general well-being of the Territories, including the provision of education and health-care. Hospitals and schools were set up, usually through church agencies and missionary societies based in Australia. Touring Medical Officers frequently came across cases of leprosy, which was an endemic disease, and in 1956 the Health Authority appointed its first 'Specialist Medical Officer (Leprosy)' in the Territories. While, up to this time, the Medical Officers had always advised sufferers to present themselves at the nearest mission-run leprosy home or hospital, the new Specialist Officer had the task of organising surveys to determine the incidence of leprosy and perhaps to 'do something' towards controlling the disease. It was a daunting task. The facts were that while sufferers who came to the mission-hospitals were given medicine, in the early days, for associated diseases and, in time, treated with the new sulphone drugs when dapsone became available, many patients suffered so badly from ulcers, especially on the feet, that they were likely to stay in hospital for years. With feet and hands anaesthetised through the disease the ulcers would go on recurring because, with unfelt pressures or pain, men and women would still walk on stones and cut their feet or handle hot cooking-pots and burn their hands without realising what they were doing.

Could nothing more be done than providing out-patient medicine and a safe place in hospital?

It was at this point that the Secretary of the Mission's Australian Auxiliary was challenged by a missionary on furlough. Should not the Auxiliary do something 'practical' in its own area as well as raising money and staff to serve countries much further away? As a first response enquiries were made of thirteen leprosy institutions, run by as many different missions, in Papua New Guinea. The replies were depressingly similar.

'. . . 400 patients in our hospital . . . the majority for many years . . . cannot discharge them because of their ulcer problems.'

'. . . most of our 200 patients have deformities . . .'

'. . . apart from giving out medicine to our 180 patients we don't seem able to do much more for them.'

The leprosy hospitals clearly needed a new injection of hope – and they had no idea where to turn for it. It was at this point, in 1962, that The Leprosy Mission stepped tentatively into the situation. Knowing that skills existed and were being used in other parts of the world which were still unfamiliar in the Pacific the Mission invited Dr Paul Brand, who had pioneered remedial surgery on hands and feet, in particular, to visit Papua New Guinea. He did so, and his tour lasted six weeks. He was horrified by the deformities he found. 'I have never seen so much destruction and deformity of hands and feet in an equivalent number of patients before . . . even those patients who had advanced and severe destruction of their feet are walking freely on their feet, although the ulcers had in most cases been covered with dressings and bandages. . . . The anti-leprosy problem is being tackled as well as possible in such difficult terrain – but *nothing whatever is being done about ulcers and the destruction of feet.*'

Nothing was being done for one reason – hardly anybody knew anything *could* be done.

'The mental picture is still with me', wrote Dr Brand, 'of patients literally walking their feet right off and finally using the end of their leg-bones to walk on!'

Now, at last, something *would* be done.

In 1965 The Leprosy Mission sent to the Research and Training Centre at Karigiri, with which it was very closely associated, a small group of leprosy workers to train in south India for specialised service in Papua New Guinea. Internationalism was by this time one of the foundations of the Mission's service. The workers were a very mixed group – a government surgeon from PNG, a physiotherapist from New Zealand and a theatre sister who had begun her work in England. Immensely excited by all they saw and enthralled by the new techniques they learned, which had been pioneered by Paul Brand in this same area, they returned to Papua New Guinea with one demanding question in their minds. Would they *really* be able to begin the same transformation of leprosy work in PNG?

The answer came very quickly. The day after they landed they operated on eight people, using the techniques they had learned at Karigiri. In the nine months that followed they carried out more than 500 operations on hands, feet and faces, restoring 'collapsed' noses, clawed hands and misshapen feet. Leprosy work in Papua New Guinea had entered a completely new phase, made possible by the multinational involvement of The Leprosy Mission, organised by the Australian Auxiliary and given financial viability by a providential and generous legacy.

But, though the breakthrough from tedious hospitalisation to mobility and meaningful life had been made, it would touch only a comparatively few sufferers. A second team was sent for training in India and, based at Tari in the Central Highlands, was made responsible for the same sort of work throughout the Southern Highlands.

There is no need to detail all that followed. Like every other country where the new drugs and the new surgical techniques linked with physiotherapy came into general use, Papua New Guinea shared the relief of being freed from familiar limitations and the joy of fuller life. Not only did the Mission teams, in conjunction with government, find themselves deeply involved in Surveys, Education and Training programmes throughout the mission hospitals, but they discharged hospital patients remarkably quickly. With fewer long-term patients there were many more surgery cases who went out with new hands and feet – sometimes quite literally 'new', for the artificial limb sections of the hospitals grew into larger units as they did everywhere else.

When in 1974 Papua New Guinea became an independent nation a fresh agreement was signed between the new government and The Leprosy Mission. Later still, in the 1980s, leprosy centres were to be phased out and its treatment integrated into the general health scheme. The Mission's small hospital at Tari, for instance, was to close and become an outstation clinic while the Mission's staff would care for leprosy patients in the general hospital. Survey and out-station work was to be extended throughout the Territories in close co-operation between Mission and state. There were no restrictions on worship nor witness. The difficulties that remained were the old, familiar ones — mountainous regions, roads and tracks sometimes not even fit for cycles, much less Landrovers or cars; flooding rivers; rough tree-trunk bridges that gave way under a vehicle. Alongside these normal problems were other things equally 'normal' but growing less so — human problems, attitudes of suspicion, and resistance to change as traditional ways of life were threatened by incoming foreigners, whether they were white or Melanesian government officers from the coast regions. Nonetheless, progress has been made. Outreach in the Highlands, or by motor-boat as paramedical workers and clinic-teams go from village to village on the coast creeks, means that the disease is brought a little more under control. To all this, working with established churches and mission agencies, The Leprosy Mission goes on contributing personnel, skills and faith to the changing scene.

Even amid all the changes there were times when patients remained in the hospital. One of them as the annual Report told, was Tomlibogo. The place was Tari, with some thirty people, men in one group, women and children in the other, sitting on the Mission's hospital verandah in the early morning, listening with deep attention to an old man with a felt hat on his head and a Bible in his hand.

Tomlibogo had discovered that he had leprosy when he was about twelve. He disregarded advice that he should go to Tari and instead followed the way of his people, sacrificing two pigs to appease the spirits. Then, when the disease had got much worse, he came at last to the hospital where he was given food and shelter, treatment for his leprosy, wood for his fire — and peace for his soul. More than this, he was taught to read and write. True, there was not much to read, except the Bible . . . but, said Tomlibogo, who would need more than the Bible when that was the place one could meet Jesus? There on the verandah in the early mornings this old, cured but still disabled man shared his discoveries about Jesus and led others to share his own joy.

Indonesia, too, is part of Australia's 'Near North', for the other half of the great island containing Papua New Guinea is Irian Jaya, itself part of Indonesia – a complex of some three thousand islands, three thousand miles in length, the fifth most populous country in the world. There are Hindus in Bali, Chinese Buddhists in the larger cities, small but growing numbers of Christians especially in Sumatra, though ninety per cent of the population are Muslim. Religious liberty is, however, written into the constitution.

The Mission had had a brief contact with a missionary in what was then the Dutch East Indies in its very early days but it was a temporary act of support. Only in 1969 was an agreement signed between the Indonesian government giving The Leprosy Mission authority to enter the country. The permission was first taken up by a small team at a hospital in Sitanala (Java), then in Medan (Sumatra) which became the busiest of the three bases, and finally to Biak (Irian Jaya). More recently Manokwari, Ujung Pandang and Cirebon have been added. The government leprosy service had long been at work though the 30,000 patients under treatment were probably a small proportion of those suffering from the disease.

The Mission personnel was international, with diverse skills in surgery, paramedical work, and experience in training and in the various forms of outreach through clinics, surveys, education and out-patient treatment. At Sitanala, not far from Jakarta in Java, there was already a government leprosy hospital and TLM workers were given visas so that they could demonstrate new and different treatments in the one ward which they 'took over'. 'The work', wrote one of the team, 'got off to a really good start, with enthusiastic support from government officials . . . lectures to fifth year medical students and nurses . . . and an invitation to lecture at the physiotherapy school in the university next year'.

Fifteen years later there was considerable strength from national workers supported by the Mission, while expatriates from Australia and New Zealand, Finland, Holland, France and Great Britain and Ireland were undertaking very much the same work they might have been involved in any of the other countries where the Mission was in action.

26: From Small Beginnings – Thailand and Korea (1960s onwards)

This glance at both Thailand and Korea is concerned with the way the Mission's work has developed over the past couple of decades, but in both countries its beginnings, small though they were, go back a very long way indeed.

In Thailand the beginnings were found in the days when Wellesley Bailey was fully in control of all that happened, responding to needs as he saw them on his tours. In Chiengmai, for instance, now very much a tourist centre, there was a plaque on one of the women's wards at the McKean hospital stating that it had been erected by 'the Washington City Auxiliary of the Mission to Lepers, 1914' ... a different world, with different terms and a different association between Britain and America! The McKean Hospital of which it was a part had been started by American Presbyterians in 1906. Through the long, lean years when hope of cure was minimal the work of compassion had gone on, with leprosy sufferers finding refuge there. With the new drugs that situation changed. But one thing remained constant, the commitment of Mission workers, both foreign and national, to the Gospel. So, not long ago, one of the Reports told of Mr Im, a Buddhist who had found Christ in the time he was being treated at Manoram hospital and how, on his return home, he invited some of the staff to visit him.

'The change in his life meant a change in his home, too ... we found all his family, with friends, and neighbours, invited in for a meal with us . . . but for a Christian service first!' As he was the only Christian in the village 'we provided him with a cassette-tape-player and new Christian cassettes from time to time.'

That last reference brings Thailand's leprosy work and its evangelism, too, into the contemporary world. The change in atmosphere and activity is seen very clearly in the more recent reports which take for granted that patients are normally likely to be in hospital only for reconstructive surgery and post-operational therapy, and that most of the work will be done where the people themselves are, in the towns and villages. There is a change in responsibility, too. With government health departments much more active in leprosy work a great deal of the field work at Manoram, for instance, has been handed over to the government health services. It is notable, nevertheless, that many of those employed in the clinics and surveys were previously workers with The Leprosy Mission, in which they were trained and gained their experience. A different transition has taken place at Chiengmai. McKean hospital, now owned and run by the Church of Christ in Thailand – like so many 'mission projects' which all over the world have been handed over to the national churches – became the subject of government/church negotiations. It is now the leprosy referral centre for all Central Thailand and the base for mobile control clinics, surveys and health education. Linked with the hospital was a child-education and child-welfare programme which gave regular help and service to some 800 children.

These sorts of changes might bring dramatic transformation to the Mission's workers as well. One of them, an Australian nurse who had already served in Papua New Guinea at the time when reconstructive surgery was introduced there, found herself in charge of the vocational department at McKean which produced wood-carving and lacquer-work for sale to tourists in the hospital gift-shop. She assisted in the occupational therapy department, and began a hairdressing course for leprosy sufferers who, after drug therapy, would need some new professional skills when they returned to ordinary life. She wrote books and edited a magazine, conducted organised parties round the hospital (a far cry from the 'never go near leprosy' terrors!), and ran a communications programme in which were prepared radio-scripts, audio-visual material and health education materials, and where people were trained in more effective ways of communication. She also, needless to say, worked in the town's leprosy clinics.

Leprosy Mission workers have to use a wide variety of skills – and in doing so discover others they did not know they possessed.

Korea, like Thailand, goes back to the 'early days'. Leprosy work was active there, and supported by The Mission to Lepers in India and the East, within thirty years of Wellesley Bailey's first meeting in Dublin. Comparatively quickly the work spread into many parts of south Korea, with small homes and refuges for 'hopeless' sufferers. Some of these homes grew into large institutions and, although the work was interrupted by World War II and by the Korean war in the 1950s, it continued to establish itself as a major relief agency up to and after the coming of DDS drugs and their remarkable successes. In time, the Korean government itself, following a series of political upheavals, began to take considerable interest in leprosy work – though the work supported by The Leprosy Mission had in fact been closely associated with official medical work in Taegu for a considerable time. The Leprosy Mission ceased to be a 'foreign agency' in 1975 under an agreement with government and was accepted as 'a national institution' – a considerable advantage to both nation and mission. At the same time several of its workers, both Korean and foreign, were decorated and presented with special tokens of appreciation of their work for Korean leprosy sufferers. The association between Mission and the official medical services was demonstrably clear in Taegu, for the Mission's hospital had been built, at the suggestion of Korean medical authorities, on the same compound as the University Medical College and its own general hospital. This arrangement meant that medical students who might otherwise pass through their training without any close experience of leprosy did, in fact, come into intimate contact with the disease and all the modern treatments associated with it.

It was fortunate, nevertheless, that the Mission extended its work into the city of Taegu itself, with special work for children and the initiation of a town clinic, for very recently the Medical School's hospital became an institution of the city itself and, as a result, The Leprosy Mission found it had to vacate its own hospital on the site.

At the same time as government took an increasing interest, so the leprosy work was more and more supported by the church itself. One of the very remarkable phenomena of the last couple of decades has been the startling growth of the Christian Church in Korea, in all the various denominations. It is very significant that its evangelical stance has been parallelled by a commitment to social justice and a firm stand against abuses of human rights. Compassion for leprosy sufferers through the years is an early demonstration of this dual nature of the Gospel as seen in the Korean church.

While in the three other areas glanced at in the last chapter and the present one – Papua New Guinea, Indonesia and Thailand – there is a noticeable use of international personnel in the Mission's leprosy work the position is quite different in Korea. There the work is totally in the hands of Korean Christians with no foreign staff at all. 'The Jesus Clinic in Daegu (Taegu) is now in full operation with a high bed-occupancy rate and a very successful and trouble-free integration into the local community', says the latest report available. It goes on to speak of able leadership and a team of keen Christian and professionally competent people.

Those who first established leprosy work in Korea and others who have known it through the years would not be surprised at the abilities, the compassion or the Christian faith of those who witness in this healing ministry. One of the treasured stories of the Korean church goes back to the time of the Korean war and underlines the effect of this kind of caring love.

For nine years Pastor Yung Sik Rhee was chaplain of the Taegu leprosy home, ministering to the thousand patients and their families, and building up a strong and virile church. During World War II, when his patients were dispersed, he was in Japan, and served in a school for the blind and deaf. Then, the war over, he returned to Korea with a plan for building a similar school in his own country. The dream was shattered by the Korean War in the 1950s and, during the Communist invasion of South Korea he was captured and imprisoned. After a 'rigged' trial he was condemned to death as 'a running dog of the imperialists' because he was not only a Christian but an ordained minister.

Taken out to be shot he asked if he might pray before he died and the surprised officer agreed. Pastor Rhee knelt and prayed aloud, for those who would soon kill him as well as for the people he loved. As he did so a member of the firing squad came forward to the officer in charge. It was a daring thing to do.

'I know this man, captain. He was chaplain at the prison in Taegu when I was there. He was good to all of us. He's no imperialist. He treated us all kindly, and all alike.'

The officer pulled Pastor Rhee to his feet and asked if it were true. It was an opportunity for Christian witness such as he had never hoped for, and he took it with joy. After that it would not matter if he were shot; he had been able to speak for Jesus to the Communists. But he was *not* shot.

'You'd better run for your life', said the captain. And Pastor Rhee did so, expecting a bullet in his back with every step he took.

There were no shots. Pastor Rhee went free and lived on. His Taegu 'Lighthouse Project' for blind and deaf children, with its factories and farm, were only part of the legacy this man who cared for leprosy sufferers and handicapped people, built up in the name of his Lord.

27: Working Together
(1960s onwards)

The date at the head of this chapter is deceptive. 'Working Together' has always been a part of the Mission's policy and practice. It does, however, indicate how particularly this factor is an inescapable one in contemporary society. In our modern world it is almost impossible for an organisation of any real significance to be self-sufficient. In particular, the greater the vision and commitment of a humanitarian enterprise the more inevitable it becomes that such togetherness is part of its life. Where the participants and the motive are to any great extent Christian 'doing things together' is today more natural than ever it was.

The Leprosy Mission crosses frontiers, both national and denominational, every day of the year by both people and by money. Of course divisions exist but important though these physical, religious or cultural frontiers may be, they are less significant than the things that are shared – the fellowship, the resources, the service more effectively rendered and, for many people, the richer experience of God in Christ.

Within the limitation that it was a Protestant mission founded in a not very ecumenical age The Leprosy Mission from its foundation ignored many of the barriers of its time. In the early days, before it had any hospitals of its own, Wellesley Bailey – an Irishman employed first by an American and then a Scottish missionary society – used part of the funds sent to him to help a Church of England missionary and then a German Lutheran. A little later Methodist missions in Burma and then an American missionary with no funds to support her, were added to the list. Through the years most of the recognised denominations figured on the Mission's grant-lists either with direct help or through support of their personnel who were engaged in leprosy work. But money travelled the other way, too – gifts to this non-denominational Mission came, from the early years, from people of many churches.

It is a process that has gone on increasing, in terms both of money and people. A list of churches and missions with whom TLM was in co-operation, issued a few years ago, included all the main denominations, ranging through Lutherans and Mennonites, the Salvation Army and the Church of the Nazarene, to 'Missionary Fellowships' on the one hand to great United Churches such as the Church of South India and the Church of North India on the other. If 'co-operation' means 'working together in the field' it also means wide international and ecumenical support. From the early days when three 'Auxiliaries' were formed in different parts of England the name was used for 'supporting com-mittees' much of whose responsibility was fund-raising. The little groups in England were quickly followed by the more important 'Indian Auxiliary', and that by others in Canada, America, Australia and New Zealand. The old name has gone. Now they are 'National Councils' and have a vital role to play. It has already been shown how much the Hong Kong leprosy work on the island of Hay Ling Chau was dependent on the support in money, prayer and active social concern of the Hong Kong Auxiliary. A number of European countries now have their own commitment to the Mission's annual budget, and equally they have personal stakes in the work going on in Asia, the Pacific and Africa.

Some of the most revealing pages in the Mission's regular magazine, *New Day*, have a general heading – 'On The Move'; and another, 'On The Job'. They regularly include items like: 'Dutch nurse after training in South India at Salur, now settling in at Chiengmai in Thailand.' 'French worker going to Indonesia'. 'Irish physiotherapist, finished training at

Addis Ababa, Ethiopia, joining staff at Karigiri, India.' 'A Spanish nurse at Irian Jaya, (Indonesia)'. And, on a more personal note, 'Swedish nurse from Bhutan marries Australian technician from Salur, India.'

The great majority of the Mission's 2,500 workers are nationals of the country in which they are at work but expatriate workers of many skills – doctors and surgeons, physiotherapists and nurses, for example – at present on The Leprosy Mission's appointment list, represent almost twenty different countries. They are not merely skilled 'professionals', however. The heading on this list is *'Missionary Staff'* – and that means not only people who 'work for a mission'. It means that they are men and women of many nations and many churches who are working together because they themselves know that they *have* a mission. They are where they are because they love Jesus, because they want to commend him and want to serve those who are in need in his name.

For such a caring and humanitarian enterprise as The Leprosy Mission 'working together' takes it across much more than denominational boundaries. It has already been demonstrated in earlier chapters that it involves working with governments, too. That such co-operation can be achieved, with trust on both sides, has been pointed out in the cases of Buddhist, once 'closed' countries like Nepal and Bhutan. Thailand and Korea are strong-holds of Buddhism, too, but in those lands the Mission has been welcome for a long time, though in both of them the depth of shared health care has been much increased in later years. After the initial delays, not uncommon where decisions have to be taken by government departments, the same kind of practical co-operation was found in Indonesia, a Muslim country with a very open attitude to religious freedom.

Perhaps the most striking example of frontiers being opened to the Mission occurred in 1985. Until recently there had been little information about leprosy work in China, though there was evidence from Chinese people crossing into

148

Hong Kong that leprosy in China was being treated with dapsone. The new government, after the end of the 'Cultural Revolution', had begun to take the leprosy situation much more seriously at the same time as it was establishing new relationships with American and western powers. One result of the new freedom was that there were contacts between Chinese leprosy specialists and The Leprosy Mission in London, and this was followed by a visit to China by the Director of TLM for Africa and East Asia. Then, in November 1985, a group of the most senior administrative and medical staff of TLM were invited by the People's Republic of China to share in the inauguration of the China Leprosy Association. The event stands out as a remarkable example of frontiers crossed and the initiation of a new partnership in the future.

There is partnership, too, with other agencies and organisations which have a world-wide social concern. A fairly recent example is in Indonesia, at Watampone in Sulawesi, a new 'station' for TLM. The two nurses, Australian and Finnish, had been working in two quite diverse parts of this three-thousand-mile-long country. Now, they were to be in an area with some 600,000 people with a leprosy-incidence higher than most parts of Indonesia where there could well be 10,000 people suffering from the disease or in danger of it – with the kind of stigma and consequent rejection which is still typical in many parts of the world. Their work would be with the leprosy control scheme, assisting and advising Indonesian medical staff surveying new areas, searching for new cases of leprosy and arranging for treatment – and in particular concentrating on schools and colleges and examining children for early signs of leprosy. The concern with children is very natural when it is realised that *this* joint action is by The Leprosy Mission, who would provide the staff and the Danish Save the Children Fund who would provide accommodation, vehicles, medical supplies and so on.

The leprosy problem is world-wide, although it is largely

found in tropical and sub-tropical areas of Asia, the Pacific, Africa and Latin America. Governments and health authorities have an immense task as they try to tackle their own problem even when they are helped by money and expertise from outside the 'leprosy areas'. But despite the often close co-operation of governments, social agencies and church-based societies something more was needed – something which would provide permanent co-ordination of knowledge and effort. From time to time the great Leprosy Congresses offered a forum for the exchange of information of every kind, but they still did not take the place of a continuing body.

The need was met when the International Federation of Anti-Leprosy Associations was founded in Bern, Switzerland, in 1966. Known as ILEP it mainly grouped together twenty-five national leprosy associations belonging to twenty industrialised countries. These associations were at work in more than eighty countries where leprosy is endemic, with 600 centres and projects. The basic work of ILEP is 'co-ordination'. Each member is able to know, and be fully informed, if they wish, about the work other members are doing; and they are thus able to share in the work of other Associations if they are willing and able. Not only was The Leprosy Mission a founder-member of ILEP but the Mission's International Director has been its President. Few letter-headings could pay greater tribute to the standing of The Leprosy Mission than that of ILEP.

There is one other element in this pattern of working together which must be singled out.

In 1877, three years after Wellesley Bailey had founded The Mission to Lepers in India, there was a gift from St John's Episcopal Church, Elizabeth, New Jersey, USA. It was very small – in English money the equivalent of £2 from the Church and £1 10s 0d from the Sunday school. No one now knows why it was sent, but it was the first gift to the Mission from the American continent. Over the next ten years occasional gifts were received though, as an account of it says, 'it is difficult to separate USA contributions from Canadian ones as all were noted as "from North America"'! The differentiation really began in 1894 when a gift of £12 14s 1d came from the USA. It included a special gift of £4 1s 0d from a Chinese Sunday school for work in China. Contributions did not rise at all sharply, and remained at about £1,000 for some years. Perhaps the greatest stimulus came from two men of considerable distinction – one from India, Dr Sam Higginbotham, founder of the great Agricultural Settlement at Naini in North India; the other, Dr William Schieffelin who was to be remembered through the years when his name was given to the Research Institute at Karigiri in south India. By 1911 there was a full-time secretary who was commended with great warmth by the Mission to Lepers in Britain. By 1920 the American 'Auxiliary' was sending nearly £20,000 a year to support the Mission's work.

By that time, however, the Americans were beginning to think it better to establish their own organisation than to continue indefinitely to support a Mission operating out of London. The decision was inevitable. The American Mission to Lepers was established and incorporated in 1920, and gradually increased its own responsibilities both in Asia and Africa while for many years it shared a 'co-operative budget' with the British-based Mission for some of the work in India.

As American Leprosy Missions they are now totally independent. Independence does not, of course, mean isolation. Though the co-operative budget no longer operates there is warm and friendly co-operation in other ways for 'competition' has no place in the service of leprosy sufferers or in the struggle to find ways of controlling the disease.

The most notable joint-action project, however, goes back some forty years for though the Research Institute at Karigiri was not opened until the 1950s the suggestion was first made and discussed between the American and British Missions as history was emerging from one of its darkest periods in 1946.

28: Joint Action at Karigiri (1953 onwards)

The Americans had long been interested in the Vellore Christian Hospital and its associated Medical College, not least because its outstanding creator, Dr Ida Scudder, was an American missionary. At the same time they were beginning to feel a new interest in leprosy research and it seemed suitable to link the two things together. In 1946 the American Mission to Lepers (soon to change its name to the American Leprosy Mission) offered a large grant to establish a research centre at Vellore. Two years later land was acquired not at Vellore itself but at Karigiri. a village some ten miles away. In 1952 the American Mission sent a grant of £20,000 to London and in September Dr Ida Scudder cut the first sod. By 1953 the hospital was completed.

But it was not 'just another hospital'. Two things were special about it and both were indicated in its title. It bore the name of the distinguished doctor who had for so long taken the lead in American leprosy affairs, and it was established, in particular, to forward research and to undertake specialised training of leprosy workers. It would become known through the years simply as 'Karigiri', but its full title is 'The Schieffelin Leprosy Research and Training Centre'.

Dr William Jay Schieffelin, the first President of the American Leprosy Mission, died at the age of eighty-nine in 1955. He had lived long enough to see one of his dreams come true, and he would have rejoiced that TLM and the American Missions have, from the beginning, met the maintenance cost of the Institute in more or less equal shares.

The implication of 'research' in the institution's title was not directed towards the laboratory but to much more practical fields. It was the work of Paul Brand in pioneering reconstructive surgery for hands and feet, and the work of the New Life village where patients were trained in village crafts, that provided the inspiration for much that would be done at Karigiri. The 'research' would be more directed to finding ways of rehabilitating leprosy patients than to experiments to find new or better drugs. The 'training' would be of those who were dealing with leprosy sufferers.

In 1966 the Karigiri report spoke of the effectiveness of DDS but its main emphasis was on 're-education . . . it has become the theme of the entire rehabilitation programme.' Dr Job's description does not sound very much like traditional hospital life! 'We now have a unit for re-educating women in cooking, re-educating farmers in farming, weavers for weaving and carpenters for their own craft. They are given a new orientation to their work. They are taught to use their anaesthetic hands with care and their paralysed hands with better efficiency. They are helped to acquire new movements with the surgically transplanted muscles, so that they may do the work they used to do in a slightly modified way.' The doctor's picture will sound familiar to those who deal with handicapped people, or those who have suffered from strokes, but it was a new and exciting technique in the 1960s to those who found leprosy sufferers with restored hands that they could not properly control or feet that would easily be injured, though they had been made new, because they could not feel the cuts and pressures in the roads or the fields. So, following up another concern of Paul Brand's in the New Life village, a special shoe-making department was established to provide custom-built sandals fitted to each patient's needs.

Specialised medical research was not neglected. By 1970 Karigiri could speak of 'research continuing in . . . the transmission of the disease, the cultivation of the bacillus, the occurrence of deformity, aspects of the pathology of leprosy' (using the electron microscope installed by the Mission in Vellore). 'Field work' went on, too. Since its inception from Karigiri, SET had ensured that there had been an unremitting examination programme in its immediate district and that, as a result, more people were being treated every year, many of them discovered in the early stages of the disease – 8,000 of them altogether in the forty-four clinics of the Gudiyatham Taluk.

By the 'centenary year' of the Mission, Karigiri was an establishment which was known through the leprosy world. It had a mobile health education exhibit which was put on show in Madras, Bombay and Delhi. It had in-service training for Indian personnel, a course for general practitioners, in-service training for smear-technicians, training for paramedical workers who were involved in Survey, Education and Training programmes in rural India. But if these were services to India itself the Centre had a much wider appeal – both to people who might use it and to others who might support it.

What TLM and American Leprosy Missions had begun other churches and countries were eager to help. From India itself the State Social Welfare Board helped to build a workshop, a rubber mill and a weaving block within a few years of Karigiri being opened. In 1962 the Swedish Red Cross provided funds to begin outreach work in the district surrounding Karigiri, and three years later the Swedish Red Cross also built a ward and some staff quarters. German help provided the Research laboratory in 1969; 'Bread for the World' (the German equivalent of Christian Aid) provided funds for a splint workshop the next year; The Lutheran Church of America helped to build the physiotherapy block in 1974 and another German organisation provided an ophthalmic ward the next year. Holland was much involved in the provision of a hostel for men technician trainees.

'Karigiri', in short, is now very firmly on the international map. This is not only because wealthy industrialised nations are eager to give help to one of the most important Asian countries – a laudable and real response to the leprosy sufferers of India where 'modern leprosy care' really began. It is so widely known because, through it, a great contribution to the leprosy problem in many countries has become possible. Without it, a score of countries would be longing for skills and techniques of which they had heard but could not have.

The chapter on Papua New Guinea told how the leprosy work there was transformed because two groups of already skilled medical personnel were sent to Karigiri to learn the techniques of reconstructive surgery – training that seemed not to be available elsewhere. That story went on to show how, within a few months, new hope came to workers and patients alike as the newly-trained team conducted several hundred operations within six months of taking up their posts in PNG. It is a story that could be parallelled all over Asia. In India itself fairly soon after this training became available there were over twenty centres offering reconstructive surgery and post-operational therapy. That number was multiplied many times over across the world.

And it was at the Schieffelin Leprosy Research and Training Centre that a large number of those involved in such work saw for themselves what could be done – and went on to do it themselves.

A map in a recent Karigiri annual report indicates where in the world its trainees have come from – doctors and surgeons, nurses, physiotherapists and technicians, nationals going back to their own countries, expatriates serving far from home, some of them committed Christians, others devout members of other faiths, some without faith at all but still possessed by a deep concern for the needs of other people. These specialist trainees, sent by Missions, by government health departments, by charitable foundations or by the World Health Organization, came from every continent. From the USA and Canada; from Australia, New Zealand and Indonesia; from Japan, China, the Philippines, Vietnam and Turkey; from Burma, Bhutan, India, Nepal, Ethiopia and Zambia; from Europe – Belgium, Britain, Finland, Germany, Holland, Italy and Switzerland. What might seem a tedious list of names is, in fact, a catalogue of men and women, dedicated to the service of leprosy sufferers who, without them, would be severely limited in the hope of a fuller life. Sufferers, in a score of countries, will find not only hope but a new fulfilment because of the skills they have learned at Karigiri.

29: The Fight Against Leprosy: 'Mr Leprosy' (1907–86)

Dr Stanley Browne was 'fed up with leprosy', and he said so to Pastor Lititiyo who had come to ask him to speak at the annual Conference of Baptist pastors in the area. But Lititiyo, the senior pastor in the Yakusu district, who had once been a cannibal chief, would not be put off. 'We want you to tell us what you are doing about leprosy, *Banganga* Browne.'

After some fifteen years in the Belgian Congo it seemed to the doctor that he had failed to do anything significant at all about leprosy. Sufferers were still unhealed and still rejected, and the church still failed to welcome them as ordinary members of society. In contrition, after he had poured out his heart, the Conference turned into a prayer-meeting, giving birth to a new concern within the church.

Back at the hospital Browne found a note from the post office saying they had a parcel mailed to him from America. He could not guess that in his medical and missionary career, just as in the church conference a few hours earlier, an astonishing transformation had suddenly and unobtrusively begun.

Stanley Browne's story had been the not-unusual one of 'poor boy makes good', with a rather bigger-than-usual twist at the moment of success. Born in New Cross, London, in 1907, in a dedicated Baptist family he was sent to school just after his third birthday because he made such a fuss at not being allowed to go, like other children! Good at sport and brilliant in academic subjects, with a phenomenal and encyclopaedic memory, he came top in everything, and after starting work as a Council clerk at fifteen he was helped by local authority grants to begin further education for two years at King's College, London. By that time he had a double dedication – to medicine and to missionary work. Going on from college to King's College Hospital he carried off every prize possible, gained his medical qualifications, with honours in surgery and, a few months later, a diploma in tropical medicine at Antwerp, Belgium. As his tutors told him, he had everything at his feet.

Incredibly to most of them, seeming to waste all his talents, he sailed in 1931 as a Baptist missionary to the Belgian Congo and was posted to one of the five Baptist hospitals there, at Yakusu. The Congo was one of the strongest Baptist mission areas in Africa and as a missionary Browne was expected to take his full share in preaching, both in the hospital chapel and on his treks in the bush. He did so gladly.

Though the Congo 'bush- and river-people' were not victims of the stress-diseases of the white nations they had plenty of endemic diseases of their own! Everything from malaria, snake-bite and complicated pregnancies to yaws, measles and sleeping-sickness were potential killers, and the mission hospitals dealt with them all. Fortunately he was fluent in French, for Browne's particular responsibility was to train medical *infirmiers*, the hospital auxiliaries. He proved himself tireless and skilled at this, adapting his teaching techniques with understanding to the needs and abilities of his unfamiliar African students and, rating those abilities more highly than most people, he gave the *infirmiers* confidence in themselves, too.

In all his contacts, however, in hospital or on his bush-treks, there was one matter that puzzled him, when he had time to think about it. Among the sick people he dealt with were some with elementary forms of leprosy but – and this was the inexplicable element – he never saw *any* advanced cases. What happened to them? Neither his students nor the chiefs in the villages he visited could – or would – tell him.

Then one day, with shattering suddenness, he found out.

He was cycling along one of the hazardous bush-paths with two of his *infirmiers* on the way to hold a clinic in a distant village where he would also conduct a service. Abruptly the trees opened out into a clearing. Browne saw a group of typical African huts, and then noted an oddity about them. They were all built very low, and the men and women going in and out were not walking but creeping.

'Come quickly, *Banganga*!' cried one of his companions. 'We mustn't stop! This is the bad leprosy!'

At once everything was clear. Browne knew why there were no advanced cases in the hospital clinics. They were not permitted into normal society. Because they would take their share of village resources but put nothing into the community the 'bad leprosy' cases were expelled to find a home and die in the bush.

Never to the end of his life did Stanley Browne forget his first encounter, in 1937, with lepromatous leprosy victims. Not least he would recall his own sense of helplessness. These were people for whom medical and surgical skills could do nothing.

In 1939, with war-clouds rising over Europe, Browne's colleague Dr Raymond Holmes returned to the Congo from leave in Britain and stopped in Cairo to attend the Congress of the International Leprosy Association as a delegate from the BMS. With three hundred men and women from fifty-five countries it was the most important Congress up to that time, and it established the importance of leprosy on the medical map of the Congo as it did everywhere.

How much leprosy *was* there on that map? The Congo government, its tremendous campaign against sleeping-sickness virtually ended with the large-scale destruction of the tse-tse fly, decided to set up leprosy surveys in which the missions would co-operate. Browne was in charge of the survey in his own area – 10,000 square miles of it – and to his incredulous astonishment he found that he was at work in an area with one of the highest incidences of leprosy in the world!

Unhappily the attempts of the Belgian government were largely ineffective in dealing with a multitude of intractable problems, of which leprosy was only one. Their response was to follow the traditional way of the bush people themselves – segregation. There were to be created 'leprosy villages' to which sufferers would be encouraged to go – though not forced to do so – though it would not be possible to find enough space even for all the most acute cases. In the event Browne's experience was typical of the whole country. With government grants a leprosarium was built at Yalisombo and some patients under treatment were urged to move there. They were fed, cared for and given work so that their self-respect should not be eroded, but nevertheless they drifted away again after a while.

It was at that point that the future of one of Browne's most dedicated and gifted *infirmiers* collapsed. Richard, generally known as 'Dickie', Likoso came to the doctor and asked him to take some smears. They confirmed his own unhappy suspicions and showed that this splendid young Christian nursing auxiliary had contracted leprosy. Courageously he offered to go and live among the dwindling number of patients at Yalisombo. Browne saw him some time later and found that he was already showing increasing signs of lepromatous leprosy.

That visit was the first he had paid to the Yalisombo leprosarium after he had talked to the Baptist pastors' conference . . . the day he found a package waiting for him at the post office.

The packet turned out to be a small round box from the American counterpart of The Leprosy Mission. The covering letter explained that it contained a new drug produced by an American drug-company and already tried out at Carville, USA, where it had shown very positive results. The American Leprosy Mission hoped Dr Browne would see if it were equally effective in Africa.

The DDS story has already been told in chapter sixteen, but part of the significance of that story was to be seen in the life of this then unknown missionary doctor in the Congo.

At Yalisombo Browne and his colleagues talked to the patients about the new drug. They warned them, as the covering letter had done, that there might be unpleasant side-effects – diarrhoea, vomiting and so on – and when they asked if anyone were willing to try out the new drug only one hand went up. The sole volunteer was the ex-*infirmier* 'Dickie' Likoso.

The results were astonishing. Dickie not only improved but did so very rapidly, and as soon as the other patients saw what was happening they, too, began to ask for the drug.

If it was 'useful' in Carville it seemed to work miracles in the Congo. The tom-toms beat out the news through the bush. A wonder-medicine had come to Yalisombo. Things began to happen with increasing momentum. At the Yalisombo leprosarium, which had 118 patients when Dickie Likoso offered to go and live there, the number raced up to 1,000 and more. Further supplies of the drug came from America and Browne's trained *infirmiers* were needed to work in the leprosarium to meet the growing opportunities. Dr Robert Cochrane, touring Africa on behalf of the American Leprosy Missions broke away from his itinerary to investigate Browne's experimental work – and arrived at Yalisombo on a day when one hundred patients were being discharged at a special service of thanksgiving. Following a new commitment to leprosy-sufferers by the pastors' conference at Yakusu a wave of spiritual revival swept through the church.

'Stanley Browne of the Congo' became a 'known name'. World-travelling journalists like Noel Barber visited him and wrote about his work; his own articles were sought by religious papers; on furlough he spoke to much larger audiences than most missionaries could do through the hospitality of the BBC. But there were days just ahead, however, of great personal unhappiness for himself and his wife Mali, daughter of an ex-China missionary. In the Congo there was growing unrest which would lead fairly soon to war and independence from Belgium. African/European tensions emerged in the church, too. There were disagreements about medical policy, and especially about leprosy work, and even unfounded personal slanders. In 1949, on furlough, Stanley Browne left the service of the Baptist Missionary Society and began to seek a new way forward.

The opening came from the government of Nigeria which asked him to take over as senior leprologist at the Uzuakoli Leprosy Settlement from Dr Frank Davey who was going to London as Medical Secretary of the Methodist Missionary Society.

In the same year that Browne went to the Congo, 1931, Davey had gone to Nigeria as an ordained minister and doctor. Like Yalisombo, Uzuakoli was the base for a great many out-station treatment centres but because of Davey's own interest in research it became the official BELRA research centre and it was there that Davey and John Lowe undertook the pilot programme of 'dapsone by mouth' which later made possible Browne's spectacular work of healing in the Congo.

Now Browne was in the place which had done so much to bring new life through his own medical ministry. Before he left there would be another step forward in effective research at Uzuakoli. The great Nigerian leprosy colony seemed to be a cross-roads in the leprosy world, and here Browne was to be in close touch with other people who were to be involved not only with effective leprosy work but with The Leprosy Mission in which he was himself to serve. Fred Hasted, the welfare officer at Uzuakoli, was to become a regional secretary for TLM in Britain. Frank Davey went to Dichpalli in India after his term as a medical missionary secretary in London – and was there succeeded by Lykle Hogerzeil, Browne's medical colleague at Uzuakoli. Hogerzeil himself went on from India to take up another Leprosy Mission appointment in south-east Asia. The

Christian leprosy world was full of crossing paths – and another instance of it was to be found in Browne's own story. Dr Robert Cochrane, doyen of British Christian leprosy specialists, who had influenced Paul Brand to take up reconstructive surgery in India and had visited Browne at Yalisombo in the days when patients were being discharged in large numbers for the first time, now wrote to Browne with an invitation.

Would he come to London when he was on furlough to discuss the possibilities of yet another new drug?

'Its code-name is B663', said Cochrane when they met, and went on to explain more about it. '. . . been developed at the Dublin Medical Research Laboratory . . . can it *destroy* leprosy bacilli? . . . we think it may do. Will you try it out at Uzuakoli?'

That was in 1960. There were more tests to establish that it would not produce harmful side-effects . . . discussions, experiments, more research all through Browne's furlough. By the time he went back he believed it would be 'safe'. But would it be *effective*? Back in Uzuakoli, after consultation with his colleague Hogerzeil, he wrote that he thought 'it would be entirely justifiable to try the drug on a group of lepromatous patients who are rapidly going downhill.'

The new drug first tried by Browne and Hogerzeil at Uzuakoli proved as effective as dapsone had been at Yalisombo. Known as 'lamprene' or 'clofazamine' 'it is the best of the second-line drugs in leprosy treatment' Browne stated in the *Leprosy Review*. It was also, as he reported at the Bergen Congress, extremely costly.

By this time Stanley Browne was becoming too widely-known a figure to permit him to stay indefinitely even at Uzuakoli. Like Paul Brand the orthopaedic surgeon, he had too much to give and was too effective a communicator and in 1963, without in any way seeking it, he was launched into world-orbit. It began with a tour set up by the World Health Organisation to research stations in India, south-east Asia and Africa. Then after a few weeks back in Nigeria he left for the International Leprosy Congress in Rio de Janeiro where he had been invited to 'chair' a workshop on leprosy treatment. The Congress was followed by official visits to Venezuela and Carville, USA, which gave the impetus for the setting-up of ALERT, the All-Africa centre in Ethiopia. Back in England Dr Cochrane successfully pressed him to succeed him as Director of the Leprosy Study Centre based in London.

In that same year he became Secretary-Treasurer of the International Leprosy Association; an honorary consultant to the Hospital for Tropical Diseases in London; the Medical Secretary of LEPRA (the newly-named BELRA); the editor of *The Leprosy Review*. At the same time he was appointed Medical Consultant to The Leprosy Mission, a position he held for twelve years.

He travelled throughout the world responding to invitations from health organisations and governments and was honoured in many ways. To him, to the end, the honour he treasured most deeply was being a lay-preacher of the grace of Jesus Christ in the Baptist Church.

It was not surprising that he was familiarly known as 'Mr Leprosy'.

30: Out Of Africa
(1966 onwards)

Out of Africa came some of the great names of the fight against leprosy; some of the great stories of research. Out of Africa came cries for help as urgent as any from Asia, and in every part of the continent Christian missions and churches had been responding to them through the years. But it was, in fact, not until 1955 that a first visit to Africa was made by a General Secretary of what was then The Mission to Lepers. The Mission had no homes of its own as it had in Asia, but gave generous support to churches and Christian institutions already at work. In general this has remained the pattern of its African involvement. The *depth* of its involvement, on the other hand, has developed a great deal. In 1966, ten years after Donald Miller's first secretarial visit, the Mission's grant for work throughout Africa was under £50,000. Twenty years later it was well over £500,000.

From that earlier period the stories were much the same as came from other parts of the world, reflecting the changing patterns in treatment. 'Schools are being visited; patients are discovered with leprosy in its very early stages; through dispensaries run by government or church many of these cases can be easily and quickly treated.' That report from Tanzania might have been from any of a score of African countries.

Another story matched the drama that followed the introduction of DDS across the world. Bwama Island on Lake Bunyoni became locally known as 'the island of miracles'. In the 1930s the haunt of witch-doctors who had led a local rising against the civil authorities, the island had been

165

handed over by the state to the Ruanda Mission of the (British) Church Missionary Society as a 'leprosy asylum'. The patients built up to a thousand or so, and the first miracle was that anyone cared for these 'rejected' people. The second 'miracle' came with DDS, and the change from painful injections to tablets, and the rapid improvement of many of the patients. 'The wards are almost empty apart from "burnt-out" cases who have no homes to go to.'

Twenty years later it would be found that even dapsone was not quite the universal 'miracle drug' that many people believed it to be, that not everyone got better and that even some of those who did relapsed again. But for the moment it was enough that, throughout Africa, sufferers *were* cured.

There was, however, other news out of Africa that was not nearly so encouraging. In 1966 the Mission's editor introduced the African section of the annual report with the phrase: 'Africa is a continent in turmoil'. Ten years later another editor spelt it out in more detail. 'We hear of conflict, confusion, big-power politics, refugees, famine . . .' There were few African countries where there were not coups, revolutions, political see-sawing. Across the Sahel region drought and resultant famine caused increasing misery and uncountable deaths. Government policies tended to favour the 'take over' of institutions such as schools and hospitals which had previously 'belonged' to European-based missions and churches, and although this did not necessarily mean a lowering of standards, by any means, there were often rigid restrictions on work-permits to foreigners, including clergy, educationalists and medical personnel – especially where it could be shown that positions previously filled by expatriates could be taken by national workers. The pattern persisted and even in 1980 the report noted that 'constantly changing political conditions, continual food shortages, rapidly escalating prices, all produce great disparity between the effectiveness of leprosy programmes in one country and another'.

Despite all the upheavals, however, leprosy work still goes on throughout Africa. In many countries it relies on the continued support of The Leprosy Mission, both through grants for maintenance or specific projects and through personnel belonging to other churches, missions or agencies who are able to continue their work because the Mission makes it possible. In several cases the Mission sponsors workers undertaking special training courses at ALERT in Addis Ababa. Year by year the little map in the annual report continues to pinpoint places and situations in which people are on the 'receiving end' of the Mission's considerable African expenditure. Nearly twenty countries feature on that map, and a great many individual place-names where TLM money is being used. They vary from Niger, Angola and Guinea, each with the name of a single place where the Mission is providing help, to four place-names in Cameroun and Zambia, and Zaire with fifteen places.

The kind of assistance which TLM is able to provide could well be illustrated by Zambia. TLM 'contributes towards the multidrug therapy programme . . . provides a vehicle for the national leprologist . . . key workers in the Zambian Leprosy Service have been supported and trained . . . a leprosy ward provided by TLM is now fully operational.' There could be many other quotations but another Zambian 'quote' establishes the fact that wherever The Leprosy Mission provides financial help this is only part of the picture. 'Fund raising within the country continues to give encouragement as churches and community groups give financial support' – words that could have been written of many other places in Africa and across the world.

A further familiar part of the pattern occurs in Zaire. 'At a large number of centres there are now workers who have passed through the training course conducted by the doctor supported by TLM. As a result of the training of these young men who work in prevention and treatment, TLM has had a profound effect on the leprosy care picture in that very difficult area.' The activities of these young paramedical workers after training was featured in a Leprosy Mission film, *Trained to Serve*.

6

Effective though this sort of training was, however, there was need for more specialised training covering workers not merely in one limited area but throughout the continent. Asia was most professionally served by the Training Centre at Karigiri. Africa, for many years, had no equivalent.

It was in 1964 that Dr Stanley Browne was appointed a delegate to the Rio de Janeiro Leprosy Congress and, when it was over, went on to America to attend a consultation in Carville at which Dr Paul Brand presided. From his own Indian experience Brand knew well how important Karigiri's centralised training had been for doctors, nurses, physiotherapists and other specialist workers not only in India but in the rest of Asia and the Pacific. He had in mind, so he told the Carville committee, that Africa ought to have an equivalent training centre. The committee agreed very warmly – but where should it be situated so that it could serve the *whole* of Africa?

When the chairman turned to Browne as an 'expert on Africa' and asked the same question Browne enumerated three criteria. It must be in a country where leprosy was widespread; and where there was both a medical school and a university in the city where the centre was set up. Later he suggested Uganda and Ethiopia. Uganda, he thought, was politically unstable – the Amin regime proved him right – and Ethiopia potentially peaceful, with the emperor, Haile Selassie, a Christian who was sympathetic to leprosy work. Browne's political foresight was no more shrewd than most observers. Within a decade revolution swept the country and the emperor and his family were deposed and imprisoned by the new Communist regime.

With no inkling of the future the All-Africa Leprosy and Rehabilitation Training Centre was opened in Addis Ababa in 1966 and very quickly the eyes of leprosy workers throughout Africa turned to it. A little later those glances towards Ethiopia were more than a trifle fearful. Would the new venture survive? An extension to the hospital made necessary by the new leprosy work had been opened by the emperor in 1971 and Dr Paul Brand had contributed to the Centre's reputation by spending six months there laying the foundations of the department of reconstructive surgery. Despite the fears and pressures the Centre continued and expanded its work.

In an age of 'immediate communication' the full title of the Centre was abbreviated into the acronym ALERT, and few titles could have been more apt. It was 'alert' to continental opportunities and to local needs. Within a few years of its opening Paul Brand discovered this when he went out on a local field trip, and described what he found in the northern part of ALERT's Rural Leprosy Control area. 'After four hours driving in the cool mountain air we came to a little township, Stella Dengaye, and stopped at the school buildings. Here were scores of children gathered for health surveys with final year medical students from the Haile Selassie University Medical School. They were checking the children for skin diseases, heart, lung and abdominal diseases, eye problems and leprosy. One student was asking the supervisor about a newly-found patch of leprosy. Who was the supervisor? The ALERT Rural Health Officer. Who was responsible for this whole rural survey experience for the Medical School? ALERT's Director of Training. ALERT has broken new ground by being given the care of these medical students in their last year at university – and new ground, too, because field leprosy control could become a normal part of the activity of a doctor in a rural area.'

ALERT was part of a complex operation including surveys, treatment, hospital care, reconstructive surgery and post-operational physiotherapy. But its main purpose, of course, was training. By 1970, fairly early in its life, it was running a post-graduate course in leprosy for doctors. Four years later, when political tensions were rising sharply, it reported over 200 patients in the hospital, a quarter of them non-leprosy patients – Addis Ababa was mirroring the situation in many other countries with its 'mix' of general medical care and leprosy patients. There were, that year,

1,028 operations performed and over 7,500 pairs of shoes made, individually shaped for each sufferer so that their anaesthetised feet would not be harmed again by injury and ulcers.

Those coming to Addis Ababa for training were not 'beginners'. They already had specialised skills and came to discover how these could be fitted to leprosy work. In one year those who came for training included doctors, surgeons, nurses, physiotherapists, orthopaedic appliance makers, field officers, control workers . . . more than 250 of them from every part of Africa, not all from mission- or church-based institutions, and they took back with them sharply-focused skills, new insights, fresh vision.

Though the support given to ALERT is more widely-spread than in its early days, and The Leprosy Mission's share of support has lessened with the years, TLM was effective in helping its foundation. Several of the early workers were TLM-funded and a considerable number of those who come for further training are from institutions and centres in which the Mission is closely involved. The significance of such a Training Centre cannot be over-estimated.

31: The Fight Against Leprosy: One More Step: MDT (1982)

In 1982 The Leprosy Mission International – its name changed yet again to fit into its changing character – met in conference in Chiengmai, Thailand. With all the expansion of the Mission's work, the growing confidence of governments in its contribution to the leprosy problem and the long-proved efficacy of the dapsone treatment it might have been expected that there would be a measure of complacency about the gathering.

The reality was very different.

There was thankfulness for the expanding outreach of the Mission, for its support in many countries and the wide and diverse skills of its international workers . . . but there were increasing problems with dapsone, which not so many years earlier had been heralded as a wonder drug.

And, indeed, that was what it was. It had come into use throughout the leprosy world in the 1950s, succeeding the painful chaulmoogra treatment by injection, could be taken by mouth and was immediately immensely effective. It had been no false flare of hope when throughout the Mission's hospitals there were services of dismissal and thanksgiving when a hundred or more patients at a time were sent back into the world to which some of them thought they would never again return. Instead of long periods in hospital, patients could be treated in out-patient clinics, often within a few miles of their homes. Cures were real and widespread.

So what was going wrong?

It was now evident that dapsone was quickly effective with patients who suffered from tuberculoid leprosy and, if the treatment were maintained, it acted well on those who had the much more difficult form, lepromatous leprosy. But the critical phrase was '*if the treatment was maintained*'. In serious cases of lepromatous leprosy *it might have to be kept up for many years, and even for life.* If the sufferer did *not* keep taking the drug regularly – and that meant, every day – he would find that he built up a 'dapsone resistance'. The two basic reasons for this resistance were irregular treatment and insufficient dosage. Even if he began taking the pills again after a period in which he had not done so, he might find that they would do no good at all. He might well now have leprosy for life.

At least as serious, because lepromatous leprosy in particular *is* infectious, the leprosy he might pass on to someone else would in their case be 'dapsone resistant', too. He would be incurable and a carrier of leprosy that resisted the treatment which, in so many cases, was effective.

There were several reasons why patients did not keep on with their treatment, why they broke off and either did not begin again or did not begin for some time. In the sophisticated world people are careless about 'keeping on taking the medicine', whatever it may be. They develop a 'can't be bothered' attitude. People in Asia, Africa or the Pacific are not very different psychologically, even where the disease is as serious as leprosy. But that is not the only reason. They have additional pressures. Drugs must be fetched from the clinic – a month's supply at a time. This can be expensive for a poor villager who has to go by bus, and even more difficult if he has to take a day off work on the farm or in the factory. Land-labourers in India, for instance, are not encouraged by the village farmers to leave their work, and the only way to reach the clinic may well be to walk.

There is another factor, too. The patient may have successfully hidden the signs of leprosy from his friends and even his family for months – but it is impossible to hide it indefinitely if he has to visit the clinic each month for examination and pills. Even where leprosy sufferers are no longer ostracised it is the one disease above all others which seems to breed a sense of isolation for the sufferer.

Was this difficult situation to continue for ever?

At the Chiengmai Conference The Leprosy Mission considered the strong recommendation that had been put forward by the World Health Organization. Just as in the case of some other diseases, notably tuberculosis, *resistance to a single drug could be countered by administering two or three different drugs.* The WHO urged that sufferers from lepromatous leprosy, in particular, should be treated with *three* different drugs. This would counter the problem of dapsone-resistance which had now become worldwide.

It was not an easy decision to make. Leprosy sufferers would need more careful oversight and encouragement, for clinic visits could not be allowed to be spasmodic. Regular and continuous treatment was essential. On the other hand, the great advantage would be that *with treatment by two or three different drugs instead of one the length of treatment could be dramatically shortened.* It might well be cut down to a couple of years.

The other factor in the Conference discussion, of course, was money! Dapsone cost from one to two US dollars per patient per year. The new treatments would cost a great deal more – in a patient with lower rates of germ-infection it might be only six US dollars, for multibacillary cases as high as twenty-six US dollars per patient per year.

Two major questions were debated. Would patients willingly fit into this new pattern of treatment? And could the Mission afford it?

The new treatment included the familiar dapsone which leprosy sufferers would still take each day; rifampizin, which they would take under supervision once a month; and clofazimine, taken every day with a monthly 'booster' under supervision. It demanded real self-discipline in the patient, new training for leprosy workers, and a great deal of new money. To a body like The Leprosy Mission, which from the beginning had been challenged to attempt the impossible the fact that experiments had produced an answer to dapsone resistance could only be interpreted in one way. Whatever the cost, this was a new call from God.

The decision was taken, though by no means lightly, after much discussion and a great deal of prayer. The Leprosy Mission would adopt Multi-Drug Therapy – MDT, for short – and face its supporters with the challenge from God to raise the necessary funds. In hard terms, the Conference accepted an international budget of £5,000,000.

The challenges were taken up in faith. Training was set in hand. Patients responded. MDT was proved to 'work'. Supporters all over the world accepted the call for new money as a call from God. The budget was met.

Multi-Drug Therapy had proved itself another milestone on the long road to the conquest of leprosy.

32: What Do We Know About Leprosy Today?

When Wellesley Bailey began The Mission to Lepers in India in the 1870s very few people knew anything at all about leprosy. And what most people *thought* they knew was wrong. We still don't know everything there is to know but at least we can begin by correcting some *mis*-information. We can also say some positive things. And, because of the many advances in knowledge and research, we can look forward to fuller knowledge and still more effective action against the disease.

Leprosy is still with us but 'lepers' are out of date.

Now banned from medical, health and government vocabularies in most parts of the world the word is still used by people who don't know any better – and those who still use it tend to have feelings of fear or revulsion for the same reason. We certainly know enough about leprosy today to allay the fears and make the revulsion unnecessary. Many ideas about leprosy are as out of date as that degrading word 'leper'.

Leprosy is not caused by loose living. It is not a sign of sexual disease as mediaeval people, and more recently some eastern people, believed. It is not the result of the vengeance of the gods, or the anger of ancestral spirits, as many people in an older China or even contemporary rural Africa thought. It is not caused by the will of Allah, as many Muslims taught; or by *karma*, the outworking of sin in a previous incarnation, as Hindus or Buddhists commonly thought. It is not hereditary, passed on from parents to children, as even men of science accepted in the last century – though prolonged contact between parents with the disease and their children may, in some cases but not in all, result in children becoming infected. It is not 'easily caught', as Europeans and Americans have often imagined. Leprosy is not, in the accepted sense, a 'killer disease' – as for instance measles is in tropical countries – though some forms of leprosy may weaken sufferers so that they succumb to *other* diseases more easily. Even untreated lepromatous leprosy would only cause death after many years.

All these misconceptions were current until Hansen's discovery of the leprosy bacillus, *Mycobacterium leprae*, in 1873 and the research that stemmed from it. Many of them still persist in parts of the world and among people who have had no chance of learning more about the disease. Even in the medical world it took time after Hansen's work for some people to accept that leprosy is caused by a bacillus belonging to the same family as that which caused tuberculosis.

It took time, too, to realise that 'leprosy' was an overworked and underdefined word. It did not mean *one* disease but several related forms. These different forms, however, have elements in common, especially that the leprosy bacillus affects, in particular, the skin, the eyes, mucous membranes of the nose (which proved of special significance) and of the throat, and the main peripheral nerves.

The different types of leprosy depend, not on the leprosy bacillus itself, but on the degree of resistance the body may have towards it.

Not everyone who 'catches' leprosy knows they suffer from it. The infection may be a transient one which shows itself as a 'patch' on the skin and perhaps months or years later it may simply disappear. The person with such a 'patch' may not ever have had any idea what it was. This is known as 'indeterminate leprosy'.

Probably three-quarters of the world leprosy sufferers, however, have 'tuberculoid leprosy'. They have more chronic and more defined light or red patches on the skin.

Most sufferers from tuberculoid leprosy have a high level of natural resistance. It is not normally infectious, but this does not prevent it being frightening and unsightly, for the body's resistance may cause serious damage to the nerves and also cause disfigurement. Hands become 'clawed' and, like the feet, suffer from ulcers. The destruction of the peripheral nerves means that there is no 'feeling' in hands or feet, and they may be cut or burned without the sufferers knowing anything about it. The results are ulcerated feet and damaged, or even shortened, fingers.

The worst form of the disease is 'lepromatous leprosy' which is found in sufferers who have very little resistance to the germ. The germs multiply at a steady rate which results in their infiltration of the skin and produce unsightly nodules in the face and other disfigurements. Lepromatous leprosy *is* infectious. The method of infection seems probably to be through the discharge of nasal mucous though the ulcers on hands and feet appear to contain very few germs.

Leprosy is found all over the world but mainly in the tropical and semi-tropical highly-populated countries of south and east Asia, Africa and Central and South America, where those who suffer from poverty, malnutrition and disease are most liable to contract it.

There are probably some fifteen million people in the world who suffer from leprosy, though only a quarter are liable to infect other people. But, of these fifteen million sufferers only about four million are under regular effective treatment.

Leprosy can be cured, in many cases, by regular use of dapsone, though this may have to continue for many years, or more quickly through multi-drug therapy. Yet the vast majority of sufferers do not know there is a cure, and even if they did know they are not within easy reach of clinics or treatment centres. As some of the later chapters have shown government and mission agencies moving further and further out into remote mountain regions of Papua New Guinea or the Himalayas, or into the vast forests and deserts of Africa, are taking the *possibility* of treatment or cure but even there it is still true that the majority of sufferers remain untouched.

Two challenges, in particular, remain. The first is to provide enough money and personnel, enough skill and determination, through all possible agencies, to reach everyone who suffers. Geography, economics and the instability of many third world governments make this far from easy. But if surveys and treatment, especially with the expensive multi-drug therapy, were widely available everywhere the results would be dramatic. Many millions more people would be cured.

Yet that would not rid the world of leprosy.

Polio, smallpox, the more familiar tuberculosis, were largely conquered in the developed world only when a relevant vaccine became generally available. There are, of course, large areas of the world where some of these diseases are still a threat – through the *lack* of vaccine. In the same way the world may at last get rid of leprosy when the laboratory research now being carried out in many countries eventually provides such an effective vaccine. The story of the fight against leprosy, outlined in this book, is one of unremitting dedication, careful research, compassionate love – and apparently sudden and certainly remarkable and spectacular victories.

In the search for the vaccine that will rid the world of one its most resistant diseases no one can predict when another victory may be in sight.

33: Mission is . . . (1987)

Almost from the beginning it was a *Mission* . . .

At the *very* beginning, of course, it was no more than a single Irishwoman, Charlotte Pim, promising to try and raise £30 a year so that her friends, Alice and Wellesley Bailey, could help the sort of despised and rejected Indians whom she herself could hardly visualise. Friends helping friends to help the friendless – nothing more formal than that.

But, within a year or so, Wellesley Bailey was back in Ireland, on leave from India to help 'organise' these 'friends at home' into something more practical. He did not form an 'organisation'. It was not a mere 'committee', nor the committee of 'a new society'.

He established a *Mission* – a 'healing mission' unlike anything that existed anywhere else but, quite specifically, a *mission*.

Mission is . . . being sent

A 'mission' is not primarily an organisation for sending missionaries, though for a couple of centuries Protestant Christians have tended to use the word in that way. It derives from a Latin word that means 'to send'. A 'mission' is a group of people that knows that it, *itself*, has been 'commissioned' and is sent out. A Christian mission believes it is commissioned and sent out by Jesus Christ himself.

From the beginning Wellesley Bailey acted on the conviction that The Mission to Lepers in India had been called and sent out by the Lord Jesus himself to do what he himself had once done. There was a limitation, of course, in this contemporary recreation of the compassion of Christ. It

179

could not offer healing, as he had done. But it could offer loving hands, open arms, and show the sufferers that Jesus cared and that he was the way to a loving Father.

The Leprosy Mission has never lost that special awareness of its commission. It has as live a sense of vocation today as when Wellesley Bailey first created the original Mission in 1874.

Yet, apart from that conviction, almost everything has changed out of recognition. And in one positive aspect of its work the transformation is of fundamental significance. Bailey could only claim that the Mission offered comfort, compassion and the gospel. Today, fulfilling all that Bailey and his successors hoped and prayed for, it is sent to *heal*. Sufferers once without hope are being offered fullness of life.

The Mission itself, in its size, its areas of work, its relationships and its methods of operation would be practically unrecognisable to the founding generation.

In particular this would be true as they looked at its budget.

Mission is . . . giving
Beginning with that Irish promise of £30, quickly growing to an actual £600 a year, the Mission income had risen to £14,000 by 1900, and to a remarkable £214,000 by 1950. This, of course, was not raised only in Britain and Ireland. The appeal of the Mission today is very wide indeed. Its supporters are found in many European countries as well as Asia, Australia, New Zealand and Africa, though North and South America in particular support the work of its American counterpart.

Now, the annual budget of The Leprosy Mission is about £6 million a year.

The immensity of its expenditure, however, is no more than a financial indication of the vast enterprises in which it is involved and engaged.

Mission is . . . doing things differently
The size of the contemporary budget is partly due to the fact that so many things *have* to be done differently – very differently indeed from the Mission's first half-century. 'Doing

180

things differently', as earlier chapters have shown, only became possible after the general introduction of dapsone as a rapid-acting drug in the 1950s, and even more after the Mission had accepted the World Health Organization's challenge to move into Multi-Drug Therapy in the 1980s. The results included a rapid run-down of long-term hospital care, the considerable emptying of hospital wards with a new emphasis on special care for those undergoing rehabilitative surgery to hands and feet. Regular out-patient clinics, with teams from base hospitals, were set up soon after dapsone became available and then, in co-operation with government health services, came the SET programmes – Survey, Education and Treatment throughout clearly defined areas to try and deal with leprosy at its source in the village. In the context of these programmes to 'deal with leprosy' meant much more than offering pills; it involved the work of specially trained paramedical workers, usually from rural backgrounds, who listed and provided help for all leprosy sufferers, especially those in the early stages of the disease. How far this 'difference' in approach – meeting the disease on its own ground, as it were – can be effective in widely scattered and underpopulated areas, or where the terrain is almost impassable such as parts of Africa, the New Guinea Highlands or the remote regions of the Himalayas is a constant and demanding problem.

Institutions have not, under these new policies, been discarded; the difference lies in the uses to which they are put. In India, for instance, there are several residential children's units, all with schools attached, for those children who for various reasons cannot be treated at home. Large Training Centres such as Karigiri and Salur provide training in leprosy work for a very wide spectrum of people – doctors, surgeons, nurses, paramedicals and others – who may come from government services, voluntary agencies and missions in the country concerned, or from many other countries throughout the world.

There is a Vocational Training Centre at Nasik – another

example of a well-used institution, and many more could be cited in countries where The Leprosy Mission has some commitment.

If the world of leprosy treatment is very different from even an quarter of a century ago this is largely the result of 'research' – continuing experiment and discovery right across the globe. It is notable that 'research' was, for the greater part of its existence, not an element in the Mission's programme or budget. It was regarded as too expensive, as something that other people must do. Subscribers gave money for people, not for professors hidden from sight, for loving care not for laboratories!

Mission is . . . discovery

Providentially those who were appointed as the Mission's executive staff had the vision that came from wide knowledge and experience, and gave full support to those engaged in research and discovery. Most of those workers, as we have seen, were in institutions 'aided' rather than 'owned' by The Leprosy Mission.

Two examples of active and practical research, more or less coinciding in time, were Paul Brand's first initiatives in reconstructive surgery for hands and feet, moving on to the provision of individual shoes and of artificial limbs; and the experiments with dapsone as a rapid-acting drug. Two centres with which the Mission has been in close association (its financial commitment varies from one period to another) have been in the forefront of research – the Christian Medical College at Vellore, where Paul Brand was first appointed and to which the Mission donated a costly electron microscope for advanced leprosy research, and the Schieffelin Leprosy Research Institute at Karigiri where, as has been shown in chapter twenty-eight, leprosy workers come for specialised training.

Despite all the research, however, the basic problem still remains unsolved. Can a vaccine be produced which would *prevent* leprosy, as tuberculosis, polio and measles seem to have been largely eradicated as killer-diseases in much of the 'developed' world? The nub of the problem for research workers seems to be that the leprosy bacillus will not, up to the present, grow in laboratory conditions and is therefore inaccessible to long-term experiments. But few scientists will ever take 'no' for an answer, especially in the long-term research which has gone on in the leprosy world for more than a century. They are never without hope of eventual prevention as well as present-day control.

In such research The Leprosy Mission now has a lively interest and some financial commitment, not least because some of the most brilliant and far-reaching work has been carried out by Christian doctors who have had some link with TLM. But such people are not interested, of course, in science for its own sake. Doctors, subscribers, scientists, mission administrators, workers on the ground all share one common basic conviction.

Mission is . . . people
The simplest way of expressing this conviction, and the massive outreach of The Leprosy Mission, is by statistics.

The work of The Leprosy Mission is carried on in 29 countries. There are 147 centres with 7,806 in-patient beds. There are also 2,701 clinics where the Mission deals with 407,701 out-patients.

Impressive and full of encouragement as these statistics are there are other figures that are appalling and depressing. *It seems probable that there are some 15 million people suffering from leprosy throughout the world – ninety per cent of them in developing countries – and that four out of every six are without regular, effective treatment.*

All these statistics, both good and bad, are astounding. Indeed, they are almost too large to comprehend. But they are only *statistics.* The reality is put very forcibly by an African bishop in Ghana.

'*There is no hunger; there is no disease; there is no poverty; there are only* persons *who are hungry,* persons *who are sick,* persons *who are poor.*'

Mission goes beyond statistics. Mission is about individual persons. The Leprosy Misison is about individual persons, men, women and children, who are sick, often hungry and very likely poor as well.

The conviction that 'mission means people' can best be underlined by spotlighting one individual person. Under another name, or in slightly varied circumstances, he could be any one of a thousand 'cases'. But the basis of TLM's work is that they are not 'cases'. As the Ghanian bishop insisted, this man and every other man, woman or child is a *person*.

Mosalla lived in Southern Africa and faced problems which were individual and overwhelming. His first problem arose because he found he had leprosy, and the second because of the way that affected his work. There was another problem, too, to do with his own 'religious' view of life. People brought up in sophisticated societies do not easily enter into anxieties like this, but The Leprosy Mission worker, living alongside such people all the time, can usually share the fears and anxieties without feelings of superiority.

When Mosalla eventually arrived at the Botsabelo hospital in Lesotho he had already seen a series of doctors. His leprosy, still not at the worst stage, was of the severe lepromatous type which would quickly cause facial disfigurement and could easily infect other people. It would eventually be quite impossible to hide it. He had managed to obtain work over the border in South Africa, but he knew if it were discovered that he had leprosy he would certainly be discharged – and there would be a long line of men waiting to step into his job. Mosalla told the clinic nurses his story, and arranged to return next day to begin treatment. He failed to appear, then or later.

In some cases 'the man' would just be another statistic . . . one more who 'failed to return for treatment'. But it was precisely here that TLM's workers' basic conviction that 'mission is people' showed most clearly. One of the workers visited Mosalla's home and found that he had gone, after all, to take up his job over the border, even though he had no treatment and had no medicine to halt the disease. The family explained Mosalla's other complicating worry. Medical treatment would not work because the 'tribal doctor' had told him that his dead ancestors were unhappy and that only when he dug up their bones and performed certain traditional rites would their spirits be at peace. It might be hoped that then, too, his leprosy would disappear.

Even though the family promised to write to him and persuade him to come back for treatment nothing happened. It might well be that the leprosy workers would feel they had done what they could; the loss was Mosalla's. It might even be felt that Christian workers would want him back to 'free' him from his ancestor-worship and make him a Christian! The TLM workers were concerned with Mosalla as a person with leprosy whom they ought still try to help.

They now took the risky course of writing to the company by whom Mosalla was employed and the company agreed to release him for three months treatment and to reinstate him when he went back. Instead, when Mosalla returned with the necessary certification saying that he was symptom-free, he was sent back home, dismissed. Surely now leprosy workers already fully-occupied with other patients had done enough?

Instead, they went into action once more. By letter and phone they pointed out to the company in South Africa that any other employees who contracted leprosy would be even more certain to 'hide' it until they could no longer do so. By that time others might well have contracted it. Perhaps surprisingly the company accepted the Mission's point of view, reinstated Mosalla and after two years, when he was stated to be completely cured, gave him promotion.

The real point of the story is not that Mosalla was cured, but that the Mosallas of the leprosy clinics are not statistics; they are not even 'leprosy cases'. His story demonstrates that 'mission' is a vocation for people who care, and are prepared to go on caring, whatever the demands.

Mission is . . . sharing

Mission is sharing skills and sharing concern; sharing with those who differ in race, religion or ideology; sharing the results of continual discovery and research; sharing the individual's anxieties, fears and triumphs. All this contributes to healing of mind as well as body.

Yet, from the beginning, The Leprosy Mission believed it was sent to share more than this. Into its constitution there is written this sentence:

'The main object of the Mission is to minister in the name of Jesus Christ to the physical, mental and spiritual needs of sufferers from leprosy, to assist in their rehabilitation and to work towards the eradication of leprosy.'

The earliest workers, including Wellesley Bailey, were preachers of the Gospel and for a long time in the Mission's history it was taken for granted that its workers would be prepared to speak about Jesus as readily, if sometimes less professionally, as they offered what healing they could in his name. As a result they could often tell moving stories of rejected men and women who had found new life in Christ.

Today, though most workers are now skilled lay-people and few are ordained ministers, they would wish, if they could, to share the faith that has been a main element in their sense of healing vocation. In many places such witness is still readily acceptable. India, for example, is a land of many faiths and a tolerant one. Africa is largely open to the Gospel. But old freedoms enjoyed under colonial rule or influence are not always to be taken for granted under new governments, and in some cases the Mission is at work in places where religious freedom has not been a tradition. In some countries the welcome for medical workers is very real but 'proselytising' would *not* be welcome. In many cases where TLM workers are part of joint local health work overt Christian witness would be out of place.

As it has always done, The Leprosy Mission offers a practical declaration of God's compassion and love made plain in Jesus Christ. In most places this can be backed up and complemented by both public and personal witness to Christ. In others, such sharing of the good news of Jesus must be more personal and quiet. Always, love in action must speak for itself—and, in unexpected ways and places, it often leads to questions which themselves put the enquirer on the road to Christian faith.

It must nonetheless be remembered that Jesus did not always demand faith or ask for a personal response. He seldom said to those he healed: 'Now—*follow me!*' He did not often say: 'Now that you are healed—*believe in me!*' When he saw the sick, not least those with leprosy, it was enough that he was moved with compassion, that he put his hands on them and touched them, that he brought them healing and peace.

It often seemed to be enough that he shared his love.

Those who follow him are commissioned and sent out to share it too.

The Leprosy Mission sees this as its daily task and privilege.

Appendix I

What is leprosy?

- Leprosy is a mildly infectious disease caused by a bacillus.
- Over 90% of the world's population has natural immunity against leprosy.
- The bacillus is mainly spread by discharge from the nose.
- Leprosy has a long incubation period – sometimes more than 10 years.
- Three-quarters of those who have leprosy suffer from the milder, non-infectious form.
- It affects mainly the nerves, skin, eyes and nose.
- People of all races and social levels can catch leprosy.
- Leprosy is to be found in most countries; there are about 30,000 cases in Europe.
- It is estimated that there are about 15 million leprosy sufferers worldwide.
- Over 90% of them are found in the 'developing' countries – the so-called 'third world'.
- The World Health Organization and the International Leprosy Association have both resolved to proscribe the word 'leper', and its equivalent in other languages, because of all its false connotations of horror, untouchability and permanence. It is cruel to label people by their disease, and particularly inappropriate now that leprosy can be cured.

What effects does it have?

- The first outward sign of leprosy is normally the loss of feeling in light patches on dark skin, or in red patches on light skin.
- The extremities may also become anaesthetic – unable to feel cold, heat, pain . . .
- The loss of feeling, not the disease itself, is responsible for the damaged hands and feet and most of the deformities which are so characteristic of untreated leprosy.
- It is one of the commonest causes of blindness.

- Leprosy does not normally kill, but maims more victims than any other disease.
- Because of the fear, superstition and ignorance which surround it, some of the major problems of leprosy are emotional and social.
- For fear of personal rejection many sufferers hide their illness until it is too late to prevent deformity.
- It is unfortunately not unusual for sufferers – including children – to be chased out of home, school, job, village . . .
- Patients are often shunned as bad people, punished for the sins of this or a previous existence.
- Because neglect leads to crippling, leprosy sufferers are unable to work; where they are not total outcasts they are still burdens to their communities.

What can be done?

- Thousands of patients are cured every year.
- Even the more serious forms of leprosy can be brought under control.
- Since the 1940s dapsone (DDS) has proved effective for most patients, even if the treatment lasts many years and in some cases for life.
- Because dapsone resistance is spreading, more effective, expensive medicines, like clofazimine and rifampicin, have been added to dapsone therapy – mild cases are cured in 6–12 months and serious ones rendered non-infectious in four days (formerly 2–5 years and several months respectively).
- Research is underway on a vaccine to prevent leprosy.
- Patients undergoing treatment are not infectious and do not normally need hospital care – leprosy outpatients attend thousands of clinics and dispensaries.
- Modern hospitals provide treatment for ulcers caused by neglect, and surgery and physiotherapy to restore movement (but not feeling) to damaged limbs and eyelids.
- Protective footwear can save feet from ulceration.
  Health education, links with local health services and governments, and successful treatment are slowly breaking down the prejudice and social stigma attached to leprosy.

- Deformities and ostracism can be prevented by early diagnosis and regular treatment.

How can you help?

- To maintain its present work the Mission needs over five million pounds a year.
- £7,000 provides a jeep for village control programmes and ambulance work.
- £3,000 covers the total annual costs of running a dispensary treating 200 patients.
- £200 provides a year's schooling, board, lodging and medical treatment for a child with leprosy.
- £50 provides an artificial limb.
- £35 pays for a month's vocational training for a cured patient.
- £10 covers a month's total medical costs for the treatment of an outpatient.
- £7.50 provides a month's food for a patient in hospital.
- £2 buys one pair of protective sandals.
  (Costs vary considerably in different areas – this is only a rough guide.)

- By your prayers.
- By a gift, covenant or legacy.
- By becoming a regular supporter.
- By telling others of the Mission's work.
- By offering yourself for medical service overseas.

What is The Leprosy Mission?

- TLM is a worldwide, interdenominational medical mission.
- It started offering comfort, acceptance and hope to leprosy sufferers in 1874, and now by the grace of God it is able to bring healing as well.
- Today it works in 29 countries in collaboration with over 80 churches and missions.
- It is responsible for 47 centres and assists another 100.
- It provides treatment for over 400,000 leprosy sufferers.

- It runs schools, rehabilitation, research and training programmes.
- It employs over 2,500 Christian workers – mostly nationals.
- While it gives treatment to all leprosy sufferers without discrimination of race or creed it is a Christian mission, and by the quality of its work combined with a faithful proclamation of the Gospel, it seeks to show and share Christ's love as the fulfilment of all humanity's hopes for time and eternity.

The Mission Prayer
Almighty Father, the giver of life and health, look mercifully on those who suffer from leprosy. Stretch out your hand to touch and heal them as Jesus did during His earthly life. Grant wisdom and insight to those who are seeking the prevention and cure of the disease; give skill and sympathy to those who minister to the patients; reunite the separated with their families and friends; and inspire all your people with the task set before The Leprosy Mission, that it may never lack either the staff or the means to carry on its healing work, in accordance with your will, and to the glory of your holy name. We ask this for the sake of Jesus Christ your Son, our Lord.

Amen.

Appendix II

The Leprosy Mission International

Headquarters:	50 Portland Place, London W1N 3DG
Australia:	P.O. Box 293, Box Hill, Victoria, 3128
Belgium:	Wolterslaan 41, 9110 St. Amandsberg
Canada:	40 Wynford Drive, Suite 216, Don Mills, Ontario M3C 1J5
Denmark:	Anemonevej 37, 2970 Hørsholm
England and Wales:	50 Portland Place, London W1N 3DG
Europe:	Chemin de Rêchoz, 1027 Lonay/VD, Switzerland
Finland:	PL 160, 00211 Helsinki
France:	B.P. 403, 07004 Privas Cedex
Hungary:	Erzsebet Kiralyne ut. 63, II E, Budapest 1142
India:	The Leprosy Mission, CNI Bhavan, 16 Pandit Pant Marg, New Delhi 110 001
Ireland (Northern Area):	44 Ulsterville Avenue, Belfast BT9 7AQ
Ireland (Southern Area):	5 St James Terrace, Clonskeagh Road, Dublin 6
Italy:	Via della Repubblica 114, 10060 S. Secondo di Pinerolo (To)
Netherlands:	Kooikersdreef 626, 7328 BS Apeldoorn
New Zealand:	P.O. Box 10-227, Auckland 4
Norway:	Viges veg 20, N-3700 Skien
Scotland:	11 Coates Crescent, Edinburgh EH3 7AL
Southern Africa:	P.O. Box 89527 Lyndhurst, 2106 Johannesburg
Spain:	Calle Bravo Murillo 85, Madrid 28003
Sweden:	Järnvägsgatan 34, 703 62 Örebro
Switzerland (French):	Chemin de Rêchoz, 1027 Lonay/VD
Switzerland (German):	Postfach 22, 4622 Egerkingen
West Germany:	Hellerweg 51, 7300 Esslingen/N
Zimbabwe:	P.O. Box BE 200, Belvedere, Harare, Zimbabwe